Cardiology Emergencies

Cardiology Emergencies

Jeremy Brown, MD

Associate Professor of Emergency Medicine
Research Director
Department of Emergency Medicine
George Washington University School of Medicine
Washington, DC

Jay Mazel, MD

Assistant Professor of Medicine
Georgetown University School of Medicine
Co-Director, Department of Electrophysiology
Washington Hospital Center
Washington, DC

with

Saul G. Myerson

Robin P. Choudhury

Andrew R.J. Mitchell

WG 100
BROWN

OXFORD
UNIVERSITY PRESS

2011

OXFORD
UNIVERSITY PRESS

Oxford University Press, Inc., publishes works that further
Oxford University's objective of excellence
in research, scholarship, and education.

Oxford   New York

Auckland   Cape Town   Dar es Salaam   Hong Kong   Karachi
Kuala Lumpur   Madrid   Melbourne   Mexico City   Nairobi
New Delhi   Shanghai   Taipei   Toronto

With offices in

Argentina   Austria   Brazil   Chile   Czech Republic   France   Greece
Guatemala   Hungary   Italy   Japan   Poland   Portugal   Singapore
South Korea   Switzerland   Thailand   Turkey   Ukraine   Vietnam

Published by Oxford University Press, Inc.
198 Madison Avenue, New York, New York 10016

www.oup.com

UK version published: 2006

Oxford is a registered trademark of Oxford University Press

Library of Congress Cataloging in Publication Data

Brown, Jeremy, 1964–
Cardiology emergencies / Jeremy Brown, Jay Mazel; with Saul G. Myerson,
Robin P. Choudhury, Andrew R.J. Mitchell.
p. ; cm.
Includes index.
ISBN 978-0-19-538365-2
1. Cardiovascular emergencies–Handbooks, manuals, etc.   I. Mazel, Jay.   II. Title.
[DNLM: 1. Heart Diseases–diagnosis–Handbooks.   2. Heart Diseases–therapy–
Handbooks.   3. Emergency Medicine–methods–Handbooks.   WG 39 B878c 2011]
RC675.B76 2011
616.1′025–dc22
2010018249

9 8 7 6 5 4 3 2 1

Printed in the United States of America
on acid-free paper

For Erica, and our children Tali, Gavi,
Yishai and Ayelet.
JB

For Sharon, and our children Daniella,
Arianne, Kira and Sofia.
JM

Contents

Series Preface

Emergency physicians care for patients with any condition that may be encountered in an emergency department. This requires that they know about a vast number of emergencies, some common and many rare. Physicians who have trained in any of the subspecialties—cardiology, neurology, OBGYN and many others—have narrowed their fields of study, allowing their patients to benefit accordingly. The Oxford University Press *Emergencies* series has combined the very best of these two knowledge bases, and the result is the unique product you are now holding. Each handbook is authored by an emergency physician and a sub-specialist, allowing the reader instant access to years of expertise in a rapid access patient-centered format. Together with evidence-based recommendations, you will have access to their tricks of the trade, and the combined expertise and approaches of a sub-specialist and an emergency physician.

Patients in the emergency department often have quite different needs and require different testing from those with a similar emergency who are inpatients. These stem from different priorities; in the emergency department the focus is on quickly diagnosing an undifferentiated condition. An emergency occurring to an inpatient may also need to be newly diagnosed, but usually the information available is more complete, and the emphasis can be on a more focused and in-depth evaluation. The authors of each *Handbook* have produced a guide for you wherever the patient is encountered, whether in an outpatient clinic, urgent care, emergency department or on the wards.

A special thanks should be extended to Andrea Seils, Senior Editor for Medicine at Oxford University Press for her vision in bringing this series to press. Andrea is aware of how new electronic media have impacted the learning process for physician-assistants, medical students, residents and fellows, and at the same time she is a firm believer in the value of the printed word. This series contains the proof that such a combination is still possible in the rapidly changing world of information technology.

Over the last twenty years, the Oxford Handbooks have become an indispensible tool for those in all stages of training throughout the world. This new series will, I am sure, quickly grow to become the standard reference for those who need to help their patients when faced with an emergency.

Jeremy Brown, MD
Series Editor
Associate Professor of Emergency Medicine
The George Washington University Medical Center

Preface

This handbook is part of a series published by Oxford University Press that serves as a guide for residents, fellows, physician assistants, and medical students. Each handbook addresses emergency conditions within a specific specialty that may be faced both on the wards with hospitalized patients and in the emergency department.

Because ED physicians have a special training in the management of emergency conditions, and because those trained in the sub-specialties have in-depth expertise in disease management, we have combined the best of both worlds. Each volume in this series is co-authored by an emergency physician and a specialist within the particular field. This approach insures that the information and advice herein is both comprehensive and practical to the settings of both hospitalized and emergency department patients.

This book is divided into three parts. The first deals with acute presentations and is designed to help you quickly determine the diagnosis and order the appropriate tests. This section is extensively cross-referenced to specific cardiac conditions later in the book.

The second section addresses specific conditions. It describes the presentation, investigation, and management of all the common (and some uncommon) acute cardiac problems. The authors have used their specialist knowledge to present the relevant vital diagnostic steps and early management plans. This section also includes chapters on important cardiology problems in which an urgent cardiology consultation may not be immediately available. This includes sections on the management of potentially challenging problems such as arrhythmias (and implantable defibrillators), cardiac issues in pregnancy, management of cardiac problems around the time of surgery, emergencies in adults with congenital heart disease, and the management of cardiac trauma.

The final section provides clear descriptions of how to perform common practical cardiac procedures. It also includes a chapter on the art of EKG recognition with a library of example EKGs to help pattern recognition.

This handbook is based in part on *Emergencies in Cardiology* first published by Oxford University Press in the United Kingdom in 2006. Much of the information has been changed to suit the style and practice patterns of the US, but of course large parts of the handbook are applicable to patients in any practice locale. We thank Drs. Myerson, Choudhury, and Mitchell for allowing us to build on the foundation they so ably established. We also thank Andrea Seils, Senior Editor for Medicine at OUP for her guidance, patience, and dedication to the project.

Finally, since this book is about cardiology, it seems fitting to dedicate it to our families, who are the beating heart—and soul—of our universe.

Jeremy Brown
Jay Mazel
Washington DC
2010

Chapter 1

Chest Pain

1

Diagnosing Chest Pain

Chest pain rightly frightens patients. It may reflect life-threatening illness: always take the complaint seriously. In the emergency department these patients are almost always triaged as 'urgent' to ensure that they are seen within the first few minutes of their arrival. The frequency of ischemic heart disease is such that it is understandably the first diagnosis to spring to mind in the middle-aged or elderly. However, remember that chest pain may result from a variety of other disease processes, many of which are also potentially life-threatening.

History

Ask about the site (central, bilateral or unilateral), severity, the time of onset, and duration of the pain. Then ask about the character (stabbing, tight/gripping, or dull/aching) and whether there was any radiation (especially to the arms and neck, which is common in myocardial ischemia). Were there any precipitating and relieving factors, such as exercise, rest, foods, or medications such as nitroglycerin? If the patient has a history of similar pain, compare the present attack to those in the past—is this as bad, or worse? Enquire about associated symptoms: breathlessness, nausea and vomiting, diaphoresis, cough, hemoptysis, palpitations, dizziness or loss of consciousness. Ask about the patient's ability to walk uphill or upstairs over the last few days or weeks, as well as any exercise that the patient does on a regular basis.

Then ask about and document any cardiac risk factors. Specifically, ask about a history of angina or coronary artery disease, hypertension, hypercholesterolemia, parents or siblings with a history of CAD, a smoking history, and a history of diabetes. Ask if the patient has had any prior tests such as an exercise stress test (a treadmill test), a cardiac ECHO or catheterization, and any prior ED visits for similar complaints. Ask about risk factors for a pulmonary embolus: These are any previous DVT or PE, smoking, an underlying malignancy, oral contraceptive use, trauma (specifically long bone fractures), any known hematological abnormalities and any prolonged immobilization, including recent plane or road trips. Review any available old records and prior EKGs. For hospitalized patients review the history of their current admission, and put this episode of chest pain into that context.

Associated Physical Signs

Unstable angina and acute MI (p. 42) Note the pulse (either tachycardia or bradycardia can occur) and blood pressure. Pay attention for any signs of heart failure. Since things can change quickly, it is important to document normal and negative findings clearly so that new problems will be immediately apparent. Record the heart sounds including any added sounds and the nature or absence of murmurs. A rapid survey for neurological deficits is appropriate (as anticoagulation or thrombolysis may be indicated) with a more detailed examination reserved for those where relevant abnormalities are identified.

Pulmonary embolism (p. 162) Look for a sinus tachycardia, hypotension, cyanosis, tachypnea, low grade fever, palpable right ventricle, loud pulmonary component of second heart sound (loud P2), pleural rub, and signs of deep vein thrombosis.

Pericarditis (p. 154) Listen for a pericardial friction rub. Check the pulse character, and measure the blood pressure yourself (look especially for pulsus paradoxus, in which the systolic pressure difference through respiratory cycle is greater than 10 mmHg). Look for other signs of tamponade, e.g., hypotension, Kussmaul's sign (where the JVP rises on inspiration) and quiet or absent heart sounds.

Patterns of Presentation

Angina pectoris (p. 56) is typically 'tight,' 'heavy' or 'compressing' in quality in the substernal area, often (but not always) associated with radiation to the (left) arm or throat and occasionally to the back or epigastrium. It may also be experienced in the right arm. The severity is highly variable from barely perceptible to severe and frightening.

- Chronic stable angina is typically provoked by physical exertion, cold (leading to peripheral vasoconstriction), and emotional stress, and is relieved by rest. Sublingual nitroglycerine will usually work within a couple of minutes.

- Unstable angina (p. 56) occurs at rest or on minimal exertion and is more likely to be severe and sustained. There may be associated autonomic features such as sweating, nausea, and vomiting. There may have been a period of stuttering or rapidly increasing symptoms leading up to the acute presentation. Sharp stabbing pains, or pains that are well localized, of fleeting duration (usually less than 30 seconds), are *unlikely* to reflect myocardial ischemia.

→ Remember that angina does not necessarily indicate coronary artery disease. Aortic stenosis, left ventricular outflow tract obstruction, and anemia are possible causes of angina too.

Thoracic aortic dissection (p. 144) typically has abrupt, even instantaneous, onset. A tearing sensation from anterior to posterior in the chest may be described. The pain is severe and often terrifying. Other features may supervene, depending on which vascular territories are affected (e.g., angina) and neurological symptoms manifest due to carotid or spinal artery involvement. The usual cause is hypertension, which may be previously undiagnosed. Marfan syndrome is an important predisposition.

Pulmonary embolism (p. 162) may present with pleuritic chest pain (sharp, localized pain, intensified by inspiration). There may be associated breathlessness or hemoptysis. Large pulmonary emboli may diminish cardiac output to the extent that syncope occurs. Ask about risk factors such as a previous DVT or PE (the most common risk factor), prolonged immobility (travel and recent surgery), malignancy, post-partum, personal or familial tendency to thrombosis, smoking, and oral contraceptive use.

Pericarditis (p. 154) may also cause pleuritic pain. The pain is often relieved by leaning forward, most likely by easing the apposition of the inflamed pericardial layers. There may be associated 'viral-type' symptoms or features of the underlying disease. Breathlessness may indicate the accumulation of pericardial fluid, and suggests the possibility of tamponade (p. 156).

Esophageal pain can mimic angina, in that it may present with similar symptoms and be similarly relieved with nitroglycerine (which relaxes the esophageal muscles, so relieving the spasm). An association with acid reflux, exacerbation of the discomfort when supine, or with food or alcohol, and relief with antacids all suggest esophageal pain, but the distinction can be difficult and investigation is often required. Remember that meals can also provoke angina.

Causes of Chest Pain

Table 1.1 Causes of Chest Pain	
Cardiovascular Aortic dissection* Myocardial ischemia or infarction* Myocarditis Pericarditis	**Gastrointestinal** Esophagitis Biliary colic Cholecystitis Pancreatitis Esophageal rupture*
Pulmonary Pneumonia Pneumothorax* Pulmonary embolus*	**Other** Musculoskeletal** Herpes zoster

*Potentially rapidly fatal
**Very common

Investigations

The tests needed will reflect the possible diagnoses and complications based on the history and physical examination and are shown in the table below. Unless the diagnosis is musculoskeletal pain in a young patient, an EKG is usually required. Remember that the EKG may initially appear to be normal in MI, PE and aortic dissection. Ensure that all patients are monitored. Radiological tests will be

Table 1.2 Investigation of Chest Pain Based on Etiology		
Suspected Cause	**Lab or EKG Test**	**Radiographic Tests**
Aortic dissection	CBC Type and cross EKG	CXR CT angiogram of chest TEE
Biliary colic or cholecystitis	CBC, electrolytes LFTs	US of RUQ
Myocardial ischemia or infarction	CBC, electrolytes EKG Serial cardiac enzymes (If an admitted patient, send a total cholesterol and HDL cholesterol)	CXR (if CHF suspected or required for admission) ECHO Coronary angiography
Pericarditis (Most patients require none of these tests, which should be reserved for special cases only.)	CBC, electrolytes Cardiac enzymes EKG (In select patients send ANA, viral titers and pericardial fluid for microscopy and culture)	ECHO
Pneumothorax		CXR in expiration
Pneumonia	CBC, electrolytes (for PORT score)	CXR
Pulmonary embolism	CBC Electrolytes D-dimer EKG (If an admitted patient, send a thrombophilia screen)	CT angiogram of chest V/Q if CT unavailable or contraindicated (will also require a CXR) US of legs

based on diagnosing the suspected probable etiology, or ruling out a probable life-threatening cause.

Once the emergent situation has been addressed, some tests will also be directed towards risk factors and secondary prevention measures, e.g., cholesterol measurement and treatment in ischemic heart disease. More detailed consideration of the investigation and management is given in the chapters that deal with each condition.

Chapter 2

Shortness of Breath

Diagnosing Breathlessness

The normal adult respiratory rate is 8–12 breaths/min, with a tidal volume of 400–800 mL. Acute dyspnea is the predominant presenting symptom of a number of emergency problems and is a feature of even more.

History

Although the differential diagnosis is potentially huge, the history often points to the diagnosis. Inquire particularly about speed of onset of the cough or dyspnea, past medical history and associated symptoms (hemoptysis, fever, wheezing, and chest pain).

Ask about the time of onset and duration of the symptoms. Were there any precipitating and relieving factors, such as exercise, rest, foods, or medications? If the patient has a history of similar episodes, compare the present attack to those in the past—is this as bad, or worse? Inquire about associated symptoms: chest pain, nausea and vomiting, diaphoresis, cough, hemoptysis, palpitations, dizziness or loss of consciousness. Ask about the patient's ability to walk uphill or upstairs over the last few days or weeks, as well as any exercise that the patient does on a regular basis.

Then ask about and document any cardiac risk factors. Specifically, ask about a history of angina or coronary artery disease, hypertension, hypercholesterolemia, parents or siblings with a history of CAD, a smoking history, and a history of diabetes. Ask if the patient has had any prior tests such as an exercise stress test (a treadmill test), a cardiac ECHO or catheterization, and any prior ED visits for similar complaints. Inquire about risk factors for a pulmonary embolus: These are any previous DVT or PE, smoking, an underlying malignancy, oral contraceptive use, trauma (specifically long bone fractures), any known hematological abnormalities and any prolonged immobilization, including recent plane or road trips. Review any available old records and prior EKGs. For all admitted patients review the history of their admission and if the patient is not well known to you ask the nurses for background and an assessment of how the patient looks now compared to their baseline.

Physical Exam

Evaluate airway, breathing, circulation (ABCs) and resuscitate (provide oxygen, venous access, IV analgesia) as appropriate. Listen to both lung fields and check for a tension pneumothorax and severe LVF. If the patient can cooperate, measure the peak flow. Continue to complete the full examination. Apply a pulse oximeter.

Table 2.1 Etiology Suggested by the Speed of Onset

Sudden	PE, arrhythmia, acute valve disease, pneumothorax, airway obstruction
Minutes	Angina/MI, pulmonary edema, asthma
Hours to days	Pneumonia, exacerbation of COPD, congestive cardiac failure, pleural effusion
Weeks to months	Constrictive or restrictive cardiomyopathy, pulmonary fibrosis, pneumonitis
Intermittent	Asthma, left ventricular failure, arrhythmias

Table 2.2 Etiology Suggested by Associated Symptoms

Chest pain	Ischemic (angina, MI) Pericarditic (pericarditis) Pleuritic (pneumonia, PE) Musculoskeletal (chest wall pain)
Palpitations	Arrhythmia (Atrial fibrillation is the most common clinical arrhythmia)
Wheezing	Asthma/COPD
Orthopnea, paroxysmal nocturnal dyspnea	Cardiac failure
Sweats or weight loss	Malignancy, infection
Cough/sputum	Pneumonia
Hemoptysis	Pulmonary embolus or edema
Anxiety	Thyrotoxicosis, anxiety. Breathlessness that *only* occurs at rest is unlikely to be pathological.

Table 2.3 Etiology Suggested by Associated Signs

Clammy, pale	Left ventricular failure, MI
Cardiac murmur	Valve disease (but beware incidental murmur)
Crackles	Early or coarse: pulmonary edema, pneumonia Late or fine: fibrosis
Clubbing	Malignancy, cyanotic congenital heart disease, endocarditis
Cyanosis	Severe hypoxemia

Table 2.3 (Continued)	
Displaced apex	Left ventricular dilatation
RV heave	Elevated right heart pressures
Elevated JVP	Right heart failure, fluid overload pericardial tamponade/constriction large PE
Stridor	Upper airway obstruction
Peripheral edema	Right heart failure
CO_2 retention flap	Hypoventilation

Causes of Breathlessness

Table 2.4 Causes of Breathlessness

Cardiovascular
Angina
Arrhythmias
Cardiomyopathy (restrictive)
Congestive heart failure
Myocardial infarction
Pericarditis/tamponade
Pulmonary embolus
Pulmonary hypertension
Valve disease (acute or
decompensated)

Trauma
Aspiration
Flail chest
Hemothorax
Near drowning
Pneumothorax

Pulmonary
Airway obstruction
Aspiration
Asthma
Epiglottitis
Exacerbation of COPD
Pleural effusion
Pneumonia
Pneumonitis/pulmonary fibrosis
Pneumothorax
Toxic inhalation

Other
Anemia
Angioedema
Chest wall pain
Hyperventilation syndrome
Hypovolemia (from any cause)
Neuromuscular – diaphragmatic
weakness
Respiratory compensation or
metabolic acidosis (DKA, salicylates)
Sepsis
Skeletal abnormalities
Thyrotoxicosis

10

Box 2.1 Diagnose Respiratory Failure

If the $PaO_2 < {\sim}60$ mmHg, subdivide it according to the $PaCO_2$:
Type 1: $PaCO_2 < {\sim}48$ mmHg. This is seen in virtually all acute disease of the lung, e.g., pulmonary edema, pneumonia, asthma.
Type 2: $PaCO_2 > {\sim}48$ mmHg. The problem is hypoventilation. Neuromuscular disorders, severe pneumonia, drug overdose, COPD.

Table 2.5 Investigations	
EKG	Think about ischemic changes, arrhythmias
ABG	Reserve only for special cases, since they are painful and usually not helpful
Cardiac enzymes	Troponin, creatine kinase
CBC	Look for anemia, white cell count
CXR	Look for pneumothorax, CHF, pneumonia

Investigations and Intervention

These depend to a certain extent upon the presentation and likely diagnosis. Unless the diagnosis is musculoskeletal pain in a young patient, an EKG is usually required. Remember that the EKG may initially appear to be normal in MI, PE, and aortic dissection. Insure that all patients are monitored. Radiological tests will be based on diagnosing the suspected probable etiology, or ruling out a probable life-threatening cause. Unless the patient is clinically too ill to leave the ward or ED, request a PA and lateral chest X-ray rather than a portable film.

Further investigations may be needed depending on the differential diagnosis:

- B-type natriuretic peptide (if low then cardiac failure is unlikely)
- D-dimers (if negative a PE is unlikely)
- Blood cultures if febrile
- Peak expiratory flow rate
- Echocardiography (left ventricular function, valve disease).

Intervention

Follow the ABC approach and resuscitate as necessary. The interventions will depend on the working diagnosis and medical history.

Chapter 3

Syncope

Introduction

Syncope is a sudden, transient loss of consciousness with a spontaneous recovery. Many adults will experience a syncopal event at one time or another, but it is rare in children. The priorities in any location are to identify serious or life-threatening problems and institute treatment, and in the ED to identify those patients who require admission and further evaluation. For admitted patients the goal is to determine if this syncopal event is part of the patient's known medical problems, and if so, to be sure that there was nothing that made the event more notable. If the syncopal event is a new problem it should be investigated as such.

The history, physical exam, and EKG will usually determine the etiology (although in about 20% of patients no cause is found).

Syncope can be caused by a wide spectrum of conditions, ranging from the benign faint to potentially fatal cardiac arrhythmias. The challenge is to identify those that require specialist management.

- 25% of the population will have at least one episode of syncope
- The underlying mechanism is hypotension due to a failure of cardiac output or a loss of peripheral vascular resistance. This results in reduced cerebral perfusion and consciousness is lost
- Loss of cerebral blood flow of 6–8 seconds may be all that is required for syncope to occur
- Syncope can occur without warning, but in some there are prodromal symptoms such as nausea, sweating, loss of balance, or altered vision
- Patients with true syncope do not remember hitting the ground.

Diagnosing Syncope

The history and examination are the most important steps in differentiating between syncopal and non-syncopal causes. Remember that many elderly patients with syncope describe the episodes as falls, often failing to recognize loss of consciousness.

History

Many patients will have had a previous episode (which may have been medically evaluated) and should be asked about their prior evaluations. There are three questions to consider, which may usually be answered with a careful history.

1. Was this a benign syncopal episode? Vasovagal or neurally mediated syncope is common. It is often a response to an overwarm environment or prolonged standing and can be precipitated by sudden fright or visual stimuli (such as the sight of blood). Other contributors are large meals (or conversely, prolonged starvation) or alcohol.

There are usually premonitory symptoms of feeling unwell, nauseated, dizzy, or tired, with yawning, blurred or tunnel vision or altered hearing. If the person cannot get supine (often because bystanders keep them upright), seizure-like twitching may occur. Vomiting and incontinence may occur and so do not reliably discriminate seizures from syncope.

2. *Was it a seizure?* An eyewitness account is crucial if there is no past history of seizures. Ask what the witnesses *actually saw* (do not assume they know what a seizure looks like). There is typically no prodrome. Frequently, the bystander will hear a groan or cry, followed by tonic-clonic movements. Cyanosis, saliva frothing from the mouth, tongue biting, or incontinence suggest a generalized seizure. Post-ictal drowsiness or confusion is normal. If the patient has a very rapid recovery, the diagnosis is not likely to be a seizure.

3. *Was it a cardiac event?* Cardiac syncopal events are also abrupt in onset and may be accompanied by pallor and sweating. Recovery may be rapid with flushing and deep breathing or sighing respiration in some cases. Nausea and vomiting are not usually associated with syncope from arrhythmias. Ask about past episodes, chest pain, palpitations, or history of cardiac disease. Syncope associated with exertion is worrying: possible causes include aortic or mitral stenosis, pulmonary hypertension, cardiomyopathy, or coronary artery disease.

Other causes. Carotid sinus syncope is neurally mediated and often occurs with shaving or turning the head. Syncope may also be due to the effects of medication (e.g., nitroglycerin, β-blockers, antihypertensives). Syncope may be the presenting feature of subarachnoid hemorrhage, ruptured ectopic pregnancy, aortic or carotid dissection, pulmonary embolus, or a GI bleed, but the patient's age and co-morbidities should be reviewed when considering these diagnoses.

Differential Diagnosis

The differential diagnosis of syncope is long, but the vast majority of possible etiologies can be easily and quickly excluded on the basis of a detailed history and physical exam. Important diagnoses that must be considered are:

Syncope with chest or back pain
- Pulmonary embolism
- Myocardial infarction
- Aortic dissection

Syncope with abdominal pain
- GI bleed
- Ruptured ectopic pregnancy
- Ruptured abdominal aneurysm

Syncope with headache
- Subarachnoid hemorrhage

Table 3.1 Other Causes of Syncope

Cardiovascular

Arrhythmias
Bradycardia
Tachycardia
Prolonged QT
Sick sinus

Structural
Aortic stenosis
Cardiomyopathy
Atrial myxoma (v rare)
Mitral valve prolapse
Cardiac outflow obstruction

Neurological
Hyperventilation
Panic attack
Seizures
Subarachnoid hemorrhage
Vasovagal syncope*
Orthostatic hypotension*

Metabolic
Hypoglycemia
Hypothyroid
Hypoxemia

Circulatory
GI bleed
Hypovolemia
Pulmonary embolism
Ruptured ectopic pregnancy
Ruptured aortic aneurysm

Other
Drug induced
- Beta blockers
- Calcium channel blockers
- Antidepressants
Hemorrhage
Hypotension
Hyperventilation
Micturition syncope

*These two diagnoses account for ~50% of all cases

Investigations

- 12-lead EKG. Abnormalities suggesting a cardiac cause include:
  - Q waves (prior MI)
  - LBBB or RBBB and left anterior or posterior hemiblock
  - Atrioventricular block (second or third degree) (p. 261)
  - Sinus bradycardia (<50 bpm) or sinus pauses >3 seconds
  - Pre-excitation (short PR interval and delta wave) (p. 262)
  - Prolonged QT interval (p. 264)
  - Widened QRS (> 0.12 seconds)
  - RBBB with ST elevation in V1–V3 (Brugada syndrome) (p. 265)
- CXR—cardiac enlargement or aortic dissection (p. 144)
- Head CT (low yield if there is a normal neurological exam)
- Chest CT if there is clinical concern for a PE
- In all women of childbearing age, order a β-HCG. If the patient is pregnant and has not had a prior ultrasound, order a pelvic ultrasound to exclude ectopic pregnancy
- Obtain a bedside blood glucose
- Routine blood testing has a low yield but is usually performed
- Carotid sinus massage

In selected patients: Echo, 24-hour tape (see below), tilt-table testing.

Who Needs a 24-Hour Cardiac Monitor?

Prolonged EKG monitoring is available in most hospitals. However, the diagnostic yield is low in unselected patients with syncope, and will be most beneficial in those with frequent symptoms or in whom you have a high suspicion of a cardiac cause. Factors which suggest a cardiac cause include a history of cardiac disease, an abnormal EKG (see above), or abnormal echo.

Intervention

If a patient suddenly loses consciousness, assess their responsiveness and check for a pulse. Keep the airway clear, give oxygen, and monitor all the vital signs. Obtain a bedside blood glucose. Most patients will have long recovered from the event by the time that you get to the bedside. The interventions will depend on the working diagnosis and medical history. Details are outlined below.

Who Should Be Admitted?

Most patients who present following a single episode of syncope can be investigated as an out-patient. Admission and investigation are warranted if the initial clinical evaluation suggests significant structural heart disease or when syncope is recurrent or disabling. Patients without clinical evidence of structural heart disease and no family history of sudden death who present with an isolated episode of classical vasovagal or situational syncope can be discharged back to their PCP without the need for any specific follow-up. All other patients should be referred for further evaluation.

Neurally Mediated (Vasovagal) Syncope

Loss of consciousness in vasovagal syncope is typically for less than 30 seconds, although patients and relatives usually report that it lasted for a longer period. It is more likely in the absence of cardiac disease and if there are provoking factors, associated prodromal autonomic symptoms, or syncope that occurs with head rotation (carotid sinus pressure). Situational syncope occurs when directly linked with swallowing, micturation, or coughing.

Investigations

- Carotid sinus massage
- Tilt-table testing

If these tests are negative and symptoms recur, then consider prolonged EKG monitoring or an implantable loop recorder.

Management

Carotid sinus syndrome (see Box 3.1) usually responds well to dual chamber permanent pacing.

For other neurally mediated syncope, treatment is less straight-forward and patients should be referred for specialist advice.

- Non-pharmacological measures are the first line treatments for patients with vasovagal syncope. These include education, reassurance, tilt-training (enforced upright posture), leg crossing, or hand grips during prodromes (to delay or avoid loss of consciousness)
- Pacing for vasovagal syncope can reduce symptoms in selected patients but patients must be informed that it does not prevent attacks
- Pharmacological agents have an unpredictable response.

Orthostatic Hypotension

This commonly occurs after standing up or after prolonged standing, typically in a hot crowded room, and can also occur after exertion. A systolic blood pressure drop of >20 mmHg after three minutes of standing or a drop to <90 mmHg is commonly defined as ortho-static hypotension, irrespective of whether symptoms occur.

The most common causes are vasodilator drugs and diuretic ther-apy, especially in the elderly.

Box 3.1 Carotid Sinus Massage

- Used to diagnose carotid sinus hypersensitivity.
- Perform with continuous EKG recording and blood pressure monitoring since blood pressure changes are rapid.
- With the patient supine, pressure is applied to each carotid sinus in turn for 5–10 seconds. If no abnormal response is elicited, the procedure can be repeated with the patient sitting upright.
- Avoid in patients with a history of recent stroke (<3 months), carotid bruits, or known carotid vascular disease.
- *Carotid sinus hypersensitivity* is defined as a ventricular pause of over 3 seconds or a drop in systolic pressure of over 50 mmHg.
- *Carotid sinus syndrome* is the combination of syncope and carotid sinus hypersensitivity in a patient in whom clinical evaluation and investigation has identified no other cause of syncope.

Box 3.2 Tilt-table Testing

- A provocation test for neurally-mediated syncope
- There are a number of protocols in use in clinical practice varying in the angle of tilt (typically 60–70 degrees head-up), the duration of tilt (20–45 minutes) and the use of additional provocation (e.g., sublingual NTG).
- Both false positives and false negatives can occur but the test compares favorably with other non-invasive cardiac investigations.
- Tilt testing is very likely to be positive in those with obvious classical vasovagal episodes.
- However, the diagnosis is rarely in doubt in such patients and tilt testing has a much more important role in investigating patients with recurrent unexplained syncopal episodes and in the investigation of patients with a broad range of disturbances of consciousness where the cause is unclear (i.e., is it really epilepsy?).

Cardiac Syncope

Cardiac syncope should be considered in all patients with evidence of severe structural heart disease, particularly severe left ventricular impairment. Syncope in patients with poor cardiac function confers a bad prognosis. Symptoms caused from cardiogenic syncope may occur at any time, and may occur at rest, although they tend to be provoked by exertion. The episode may be associated with palpitations or chest discomfort.

Investigations

- Echocardiography
- Prolonged EKG monitoring
- *In selected patients*: Electrophysiological studies
- Syncope occurring during exertion should be investigated with echocardiography and exercise stress testing.

Important Causes of Cardiac Syncope

Obtain an urgent cardiology consultation in each of the following cases:

Severe left ventricular impairment (p. 72)

Associated with monomorphic VT, atrial arrhythmias, postural or drug-induced hypotension.

Aortic stenosis (p. 133)

Exertional syncope resulting from severe aortic stenosis is associated with a high incidence of sudden death.

Table 3.2 Types of Brugada Syndrome			
	Type 1	**Type 2**	**Type 3**
J-Point	> (or =) 2 mm	> (or =) 2 mm	> (or =) 2 mm
T-wave	Negative	Positive or biphasic	Positive
ST-T configuration	Coved	Saddleback	Saddleback
ST-segment, Terminal portion	Gradually descending	Elevated > (or =) 1 mm	Elevated <1 mm

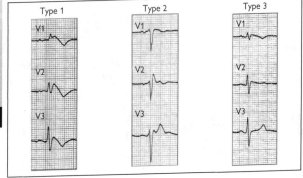

Figure 3.1 EKG pattern in Brugada syndrome.
Source: Napolitano C, Priori SG. Brugada syndrome. *Orphanet J Rare Dis.* 2006;1:35. © BioMed Central.

Hypertrophic cardiomyopathy (p. 71)
Syncope occurs in up to 25% of patients and can be a risk marker for sudden cardiac death.

Long QT syndrome (p. 102, EKG p. 264)
Episodes of polymorphic VT can result in recurrent syncope.

Brugada syndrome (EKG p. 265)
This is a genetic defect of sodium channels, and may cause sudden cardiac death. Look for RBBB and ST elevations in the right precordial leads (V1–V3).

Chapter 4

Cardiovascular Collapse

21

Cardiovascular Collapse

Cardiovascular collapse is the rapid or sudden development of circulatory failure. This forms part of a spectrum which encompasses:

• Cardiac arrest
• Shock

Cardiac Arrest

Cardiac arrest occurs with asystole, a condition in which there is a complete loss of cardiac function and no cardiac output. Bradycardia and tachycardia may also cause the loss of cardiac output, and result in a loss of consciousness. Each condition must be treated immediately, following the most current ACLS guidelines. These are shown in Figures 4.1, 4.2, and 4.3.

Shock

This is most commonly defined as a systolic BP <90 mmHg with features of reduced organ perfusion.

In shock, cardiac output may be high (e.g., sepsis) or low (e.g., cardiogenic shock). The common factor is a failure of tissue oxygen delivery and/or tissue oxygen utilization. The clinical presentation will depend on the severity and speed of onset of the cause and the physiologic reserve of the host. Determining the cause may be difficult and the diagnosis may only be apparent following, or during, resuscitation. Remember that pathologies frequently co-exist, particularly in the elderly (e.g., cardiac failure complicating sepsis).

→ Assessment and treatment should proceed in parallel.

The immediate priorities are to maintain:

• A safe airway and oxygenation
• Sufficient circulation to perfuse the heart and brain.

Once these have been achieved, there is time to refine the diagnosis and perform any special investigations and specific treatment while continuing to monitor the patient.

The Initial Assessment

This should be rapid. You need to decide whether the patient can survive more detailed assessment or whether you must start resuscitating immediately.

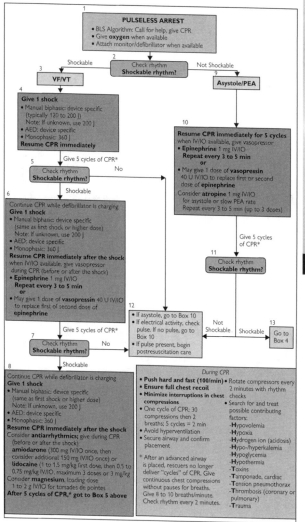

Figure 4.1 ACLS pulseless arrest algorithm.
Reprinted with permission 2005 AHA Guidelines for Cardiopulmonary Resuscitation and Emergency Cardiovascular Care, Part 7.2: Management of Cardiac Arrest. *Circulation* 2005;112: IV-58-IV-66. © 2005, American Heart Association, Inc.

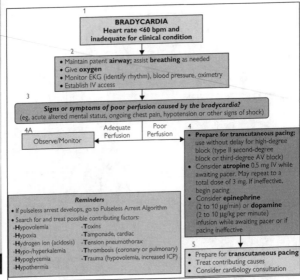

Figure 4.2 ACLS bradycardia algorithm.
Reprinted with permission from *Circulation* 2005; 112: IV67-77. © 2005 American
Heart Association. Fig. 1, p. IV-68.

→ If the patient can speak, take a brief, focused history. If not, assess
the patient while questioning nursing staff, ambulance personnel, or
relatives. If you are able to review the hospital records, do so; otherwise delegate a colleague to perform that task.

Box 4.1 Immediate Priorities—ABC

- Check that the airway is patent
- Is the patient breathing?
- Check the circulation

Specifically Examine

- Check the trachea
- Percuss the upper chest and listen to air entry to exclude
  pneumothorax and for crackles of pulmonary edema
- Listen to the heart. Are there any (possibly new) murmurs?
- Quickly feel the abdomen for distension and pulsatile masses
- Check the peripheral perfusion, including capillary refill
- Recheck the blood pressure
- JVP
- Is there a sternotomy scar?

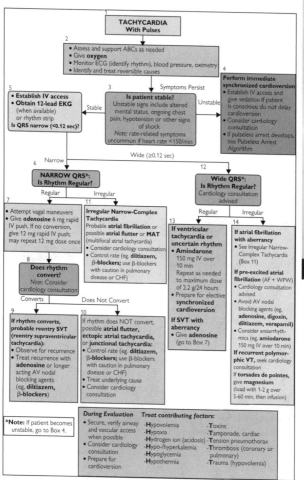

Figure 4.3 ACLS tachycardia algorithm.
Reprinted with permission from *Circulation* 2005; 112: IV67-77. © 2005 American Heart Association. Fig. 2, p. IV-70.

- Assess conscious level using the AVPU score:
  - A = awake
  - V = responds to voice only
  - P = responds to pain
  - U = unresponsive
- Check a blood glucose at the bedside.

Obtain (or Nominate a Colleague to Obtain)

- 12-lead ECG
- Chest X-ray
- ABG if the patient is intubated or there is a question about the oxygenation
- Urgent CBC, electrolytes, and cardiac enzymes
- If sepsis seems likely send blood cultures.

Approaching a Differential in Shock

By this stage you should have sufficient information to make a preliminary diagnosis and assign the cause of the shock to one of four main categories, as shown in Box 4.2.

Causes of Shock

Box 4.2 Causes of Shock

Cardiogenic

- Acute myocardial failure
- Acute myocardial ischemia
- Acute valve failure
- Acute valvular lesion
- Arrhythmias
- Cardio-depressant drugs
- Myocarditis

Hypovolemic

- Hemorrhage (e.g., GI bleeding, aortic dissection, post trauma)
- Fluid loss (dehydration, burns, polyuria)
- Adrenal failure

Obstruction

- Pericardial tamponade
- Pulmonary embolus
- Tension pneumothorax

Systemic vasodilatation

- Sepsis
- Liver failure
- Drug overdose
- Anaphylaxis

Immediate Interventions

→ Reassess airway, breathing, circulation (ABC) frequently. Treat cardiac arrest following ACLS protocols (pp. 23–25).

Airway Management

- Place an oral or nasal airway if the patient is unconscious in order to maintain airway
- Give high-flow O_2 via a reservoir bag or assist ventilation with bag and mask
- For a tension pneumothorax perform immediate needle thoracostomy followed by a chest drain
- If the patient is conscious and is hypoxic, and has either pulmonary edema or is in respiratory distress, continuous airways pressure (CPAP see p. 30) may be an alternative to intubation. Call respiratory therapy to the bedside to set up the CPAP equipment.

When to call anesthesia

Always call anesthesia if you do not feel comfortable or competent in managing the airway. In the ED there is rarely a need to call for them. However, on the inpatient floors experience may be lacking, so have a low threshold for calling. Many hospitals have a rapid response team that consists of an anesthetist and respiratory technician. Have the team paged if you need help.

Circulatory Management

- Establish good peripheral IV access
- If there is significant bradycardia, give atropine 0.5–1 mg IV and consider external pacing if inadequate response (p. 252)
- If the patient is not in cardiogenic shock and has no evidence of intravascular volume overload or pulmonary edema, give rapid IV fluid challenge (500 cc of normal saline). If there is a beneficial response, repeat the bolus.
- If the blood pressure remains low (< ~70 mmHg systolic) despite adequate filling and treatment of immediately reversible causes, obtain central venous access and start inotropes (see Table 4.1).

General Management

- If the blood glucose is low, give 50 cc of 50% dextrose immediately
- If pupils are constricted and patient is unresponsive, give naloxone 1 mg IV stat. Give 2–3 mg before concluding that there is no response. If there is some improvement, repeat the dose. If the patient has received an accidental overdose of narcotics, large doses of naloxone may be required.

Table 4.1 Table of Inotropes

		Formulation	Dose Range	Initial Dose (70 kg man)
VASODILATORS				
Nitroglycerin				
Initial treatment of angina or acute LVF	Bolus (sublingual spray)	500 mcg		2–4 puffs
Continued treatment of angina or LVF	Infusion 1 mg/mL	50 mg in 50 mL 0.9% saline	0.5–20 mg/h	2–5 mL/h
INODILATORS				
Dobutamine	Infusion 5 mg/mL	250 mg in 50 mL 0.9% saline	1.25–10 mcg/kg/min	1.6–4 mL/h (approx 2–5 mcg/kg/min)
INOCONSTRICTORS				
Epinephrine				
In extremis	Bolus (minijet)	1 mg in 10 mL	p.r.n.	0.5 mL bolus
Increase BP and cardiac output	Infusion	4 mg in 50 mL 0.9% saline	Up to 50 mL/h (titrate to effect)	2–5 mL/h
Dopamine	Infusion	200 mg in 50 mL 0.9% saline	1–10 mcg/kg/min	2–5 mL/h (approx 2–5 mcg/kg/min)
As epinephrine				

Ephedrine As epinephrine Slower onset (2–10 min) and longer lasting	Bolus 3 mg/mL	Dilute 30 mg (1 mL) to 10 mL with 0.9% saline		1 mL of dilute solution
VASOCONSTRICTORS				
Norepinephrine 'Pure' vasoconstriction—increase BP, little effect on CO	Infusion	4 mg in 50 mL 0.9% saline	Up to 50 mL/h (titrate to effect)	2–5 mL/h
Metaraminol Pure' vasoconstrictor. Slow onset—max effect at 10 minutes	Bolus	Dilute 10 mg (1 mL) to 10 mL with 0.9% saline		0.5–5 mL bolus of dilute solution

Infusions should be given centrally. Dopamine and dobutamine can be given peripherally at lower concentrations (dilute in 500 mL, not 50 mL). Caution with extravasation of bolus drugs. An inoconstrictor (epinephrine or dopamine) can be used if norepinephrine is not immediately on hand. Norepinephrine is preferable if the patient is very tachycardic (>120 bpm) or if there is clear evidence of myocardial ischemia. Ephedrine or metaraminol are reasonable alternatives for peripheral boluses.

Continuous Positive Airway Pressure (CPAP)

In left ventricular dysfunction, CPAP has pulmonary and cardiac benefits. It increases functional residual capacity, thus increasing the effective alveolar surface area and improving oxygenation and, in most patients, reduces the work of breathing. (However use caution in patients with a hyper-inflated chest or restrictive chest-wall disease). Cardiac effects include a reduction in LV preload, improved ejection fraction, and reduction in mitral regurgitation.

Monitoring and Assessment of the Circulation

Assess and continually insure that the circulation is adequate:

- The heart rate should be 60–100 beats per minute, but higher or lower rates may be acceptable if all other components of the circulation are adequate
- Mean arterial blood pressure (diastolic + pulse pressure/3) should be at least 60 to allow adequate cerebral perfusion. Previously hypertensive patients may require a higher pressure
- Diastolic BP must be sufficient to allow myocardial perfusion (>35–40 mmHg, no ST depression on ECG)
- Urine output >0.5 mL/kg/h
- Capillary refill should be <2 seconds
- Lactate concentration should be <2.0 mmol/L, preferably <1.6. If it is higher, it should fall in response to resuscitation.

Continuing Investigation and Treatment

If the underlying diagnosis is obvious, you can now initiate definitive treatment. If however, the etiology is still in doubt, obtain a stat bedside echocardiogram. This will give information about the following:

- LV dysfunction (think of MI, myocarditis, and cardiomyopathy)
- Wall-motion abnormalities (think ischemia)
- Valvular/structural lesions (see p. 110)
- Pericardial disease and cardiac tamponade (p. 156)
- Right-sided cardiac dilatation (think PE, decompensated pulmonary hypertension, see p. 162)

Other investigations might include:

- CT pulmonary angiogram (PE)
- CT thorax/abdomen (aortic/intra-abdominal pathology).

Central Venous Monitoring

A central venous line should be placed via the internal jugular or subclavian route into the superior vena cava (see p. 245). This allows monitoring of right-sided filling pressures and the dynamic response to fluid challenges, repeated central venous blood gas estimation. While this is of no value for pO_2 and pCO_2, it is useful for tracking changes in pH and lactate, as well as estimating the central venous oxygen saturation ($ScvO_2$).

Central venous pressure

The normal CVP is 4–8 cmH_2O and reflects both right and left ventricular end-diastolic pressures. Changes in circulating volume, vasoconstriction or dilatation, and pulmonary vascular disease may all mean that CVP does not reflect left-sided filling pressures.

→ In all causes of shock, the myocardial filling pressure will need to be increased to maintain stroke volume. Consequently, a static measurement of CVP is of little value and it is better to measure the response to a volume challenge.

Fluid challenge

- The principle is that a fluid challenge will produce an initial rise in CVP but when the infusion is completed, the fluid will redistribute and the CVP will then fall, particularly in hypovolemia
- In euvolemic patients, there will be a net increase in CVP which will be sustained
- Measure the baseline CVP, and then give a bolus infusion, (generally 200 mL of colloid over 10–15 minutes). Then measure the CVP once the bolus is completed and again 10–15 minutes later
- A sustained rise in CVP above baseline of >3 cmH_2O suggests that the patient is euvolemic
- An initial rise then a fall, or failure of the CVP to rise by 3 cmH_2O, implies hypovolemia, and more fluid should be given.
- Be extra cautious in giving fluid challenges to patients with severe heart failure.

Central venous oxygen saturation ($ScvO_2$) measurement

- If the cardiac output is low in relation to tissue oxygen demand, more oxygen will be extracted per unit of blood and the saturation of venous blood will fall
- A true mixed venous oxygen sample taken from the pulmonary artery reflects the balance between tissue oxygen delivery and consumption, and a surrogate estimate can be obtained from the SVC
- Normal $ScvO_2$ is approximately 80%
- An $ScvO_2$ of less than 70% implies that the cardiac output is low. If there is other evidence of tissue hypoperfusion, there may be a benefit in increasing the cardiac output (e.g., with fluids and inotropes)
- If the $ScvO_2$ is >70%, there is probably little value in increasing cardiac output further with inotropes.

31

Intra-aortic Balloon Pump (IABP)

Intra-aortic balloon pump (IABP) devices are mostly used in the CCU. Indications and contraindications are in Box 4.3.

How they work

- A long balloon (34 or 40 cm) is placed in the proximal descending aorta. Rapid expansion of the balloon in diastole displaces blood and promotes flow distally to the mesenteric, renal, and lower limb vessels
- Augmented flow also occurs proximal to the balloon, to the head and neck vessels and coronary arteries
- Flow in the coronary vessels mainly occurs in diastole. An IABP is associated with a substantial improvement in coronary perfusion
- Abrupt balloon deflation at the start of systole decreases the after load resistance to left ventricular contraction, improving performance and decreasing cardiac work
- The balloon is inflated and deflated with helium via a pressurized line, fed from a reservoir cylinder
- Inflation and deflation cycles are timed from the surface EKG and adjusted so that the balloon inflates immediately after closure of the aortic valve and then deflates at the end of diastole.

Practical considerations

Consider the following points when caring for a patient with an IABP.

- All patients should receive systemic anticoagulation with IV heparin
- IABP therapy is less effective in patients with a tachycardia, especially if the rhythm is irregular. These patients should be reexamined by the cardiac fellow or attending physician, and will often need to have the inflation/deflation cycles triggered by changes in aortic pressure rather than the surface EKG
- In the event of IABP failure (balloon rupture, exhausted helium supply, EKG trigger failure) pumping must be resumed in 10–15 minutes or the balloon catheter removed. A static IABP is a potential source of clot formation and distal arterial embolization
- IABP catheters can be inserted directly or via a sheath into the femoral artery. At the time of removal, the used balloon will not however retract through the sheath. The IABP catheter should be slowly withdrawn until the balloon reaches the sheath. At this point resistance will be encountered. The sheath and balloon catheter are then pulled out together as a single unit. Pressure hemostasis will be required as for any arterial line. Remember that IABP catheters tend to be 8F or bigger and prolonged compression of the artery will be required

- Some patients require weaning from IABP support. The usual method is to reduce the balloon inflation frequency to every second, and later to every third cardiac cycle.
- Though it is possible to draw an arterial blood sample from the pressure monitoring line of an IABP, this should be avoided as the caliber of the line is narrow and prone to blockage if contaminated with blood.

Box 4.3 Intra-aortic Balloon Pump Insertion

Indications

- Cardiogenic shock
- Intractable myocardial ischemia
- Severe pulmonary edema
- Severe mitral regurgitation with cardiac failure
- Ventricular septal defect with severe cardiac failure (esp. post-MI)
- Support during CABG and coronary angioplasty.

Contraindications

- Significant aortic regurgitation
- Significant aortic stenosis
- Hypertrophic obstructive cardiomyopathy with significant gradient
- Significant peripheral vascular disease (relative contraindication).

Cautions

- May worsen renal and mesenteric blood flow
- Peripheral vascular compromise can occur, usually affecting the leg on the side of insertion, although ischemia of the contralateral limb can also occur. A cold, pale, and painful limb with reduced pulses demands immediate attention and a stat consult from vascular surgery.

Palpitations

Introduction

Palpitations are a sensation in which the patient can feel his beating heart. The sensation is often very frightening, and is a common cause of visits to the emergency department and cardiology clinic.

History

The history will vary from individual to individual. In some it is nothing more than an awareness of the heartbeat. Others may give a history of pounding or fluttering in the chest. Find out if this was one of many episodes, and if so, for how long has the patient been experiencing symptoms? If this is one of many episodes but is the first time that the patient has seen a physician, ask what was different about the episode that led to the current visit. Ask what the patient was doing immediately prior to the onset of symptoms, and how long the symptoms lasted. If possible, ask the patient to tap out the rhythm that was felt. Ask about any family history of arrhythmias or sudden death. Obtain a full drug history, remembering that recreational drugs, caffeine, and many herbal medications may cause palpitations. Perhaps most importantly, ask if the symptoms were associated with any dizziness or loss of consciousness, since this suggests a ventricular arrhythmia, which must be emergently diagnosed. Once this history has been obtained, consider the following:

Table 5.1 Considerations	
1. What is the rhythm?	
Pounding heart	—may be physiological
Sudden one-off 'jump'	—unimportant, likely ectopic beat
Irregular heart beat	—likely multiple ectopic beats or AF
Fast heart rhythm	—consider tachyarrhythmia.
2. What is the pattern?	
Abrupt onset/cessation	SVT, VT, AF
Slow increase/decrease	Sinus tachycardia
At times of stress/anxiety	Anxiety/emotion
Related to exertion	Sinus, AF, SVT if abrupt onset
Early beat, pause then heavy beat	Ventricular ectopic beats
Irregular rhythm	AF, multiple ectopic beats.
3. What is the duration?	
Brief (few seconds)	Atrial/ventricular ectopics
Several minutes/few hours	SVT/AF
Continuous	Sinus tachycardia/thyrotoxicosis.
4. What is the previous history?	
Known poor LV function	—VT more likely
Previous SVT/AF/VT	—recurrence?

Physical Exam

Most cases of palpitations will have resolved by the time the patient is seen in the ED or clinic, and in the vast majority of cases the physical exam is normal. However, focus on the cardiac exam and listen carefully for the mid-systolic click that indicates mitral valve prolapse, since palpitations are a very common presentation of this disorder.

Investigation

In the ED, obtain an EKG and insure that the patient is on a cardiac monitor for the duration of the visit. If the patient is on diuretics or may be anemic, it is important to obtain a CBC and BMP, since anemia or electrolyte abnormalities may result in arrhythmias. Since most patients will have these routine lab tests as part of their follow-up cardiology evaluation, you may also choose to obtain them during the ED visit.

In most cases the initial ED or clinic evaluation will not result in the etiology being determined. If at this stage you think a true arrhythmia may be present, proceed with an echocardiogram and arrange for ambulatory EKG monitoring, more commonly referred to as Holter monitoring. There are several different types of monitoring:

- 24/48 hour EKG monitor: good for frequent symptoms, may need several before rhythm identified
- Patient-activated event recorder. The EKG, stored during an episode, can be downloaded to cardiology clinic over the telephone. Device may be kept for several weeks, which makes this recorder good for less frequent episodes. Of course, the patient needs to be alert during episode and capable of operating device.
- Implantable loop recorders—a small device implanted under the skin in pectoral or axillary region. It typically records 40 minutes of EKG, recorded by a patient-activated key or stored automatically. This monitor is good for infrequent but more symptomatic episodes.

Intervention

If the patient presents with palpitations and a continuing arrhythmia, manage the arrhythmia as appropriate (see pp. 76–104).

Differential Diagnosis

The following cardiac etiologies should be considered. They are in order of decreasing likelihood:

- Normal sinus rhythm
- Premature ventricular contractions

Table 5.2 EKG Clues to the Cause of Palpitations	
EKG Findings	Possible Cause
Short PR interval, delta waves	AV reentrant tachycardia
P mitrale, LVH, PACs	Atrial fibrillation
PVCs, LBBB	Ventricular tachycardia
Q waves	Ventricular tachycardia
Heart block	PVCs, ventricular tachycardia
Prolonged QT interval	Ventricular tachycardia

- Premature atrial contractions
- Atrial fibrillation (p. 86)
- Ventricular tachycardia (p. 100)
- Supraventricular tachycardia (p. 95)

Noncardiac causes should also be considered:

- Sinus tachycardia—pain, anxiety, fear, exertion, hypoxia, infection, hypovolemia (e.g. dehydration), anemia and thyrotoxicosis
- Gastro-esophageal reflux
- Anxiety
- Very rare—Pheochromocytoma and carcinoid syndrome.

While waiting for the results of the Holter monitoring, the EKG will provide some clues as to the etiology of the palpitations.

If you are working up the patient in the ED, a cardiology consultation is only needed if you strongly suspect a ventricular tachycardia as a cause.

Management

The key to disposition is to risk stratify the patient. **High risk** patients are those who present with palpitations and

- A previous MI (which may lead to myocardial scarring)
- Cardiomyopathy
- Valvular stenosis or regurgitation
- Sudden death from cardiac causes in the family
- Long QT syndrome on the EKG

All other patients fall into the **low risk** category. From the ED, high risk patients should be referred to a cardiology clinic for further evaluation. This will typically involve a Holter monitor or continuous-loop event recorder. Low risk patients usually only need referral if there is a suspicion of a sustained arrhythmia or if the patient is especially anxious to be seen by a cardiologist.

Document a careful history looking for concerning arrhythmias as outlined above, and a focused physical and full cardiac exam, showing no evidence of valve disease. The EKG should document a normal QT interval.

Chapter 6

Acute Coronary Syndromes

Acute Coronary Syndromes (ACS)

Ischemic heart disease is a leading cause of death in the Western world. Mortality from acute MI is believed to be 45%, with 70% of these deaths occurring before reaching medical care. Contributory risk factors for MI include smoking, hypertension, age, male sex, diabetes, hyperlipidemia, and a family history.

Acute coronary syndrome comprises a spectrum of clinical conditions, all caused by impaired flow in the coronary arteries:

- acute ST segment elevation MI (STEMI)
- non ST segment elevation MI (NSTEMI)
- unstable angina (ACS without elevation of troponin or cardiac enzymes)

Pathophysiology

Understanding the pathophysiology helps to explain the spectrum of presentation and underpins rational treatment.

Chronic stable angina occurs when fixed stenotic lesions impede myocardial perfusion at times of increased oxygen demand.

Acute coronary syndromes, in contrast, occur when erosion or rupture of the 'fibrous cap' overlying an atherosclerotic lesion exposes intensely thrombogenic material within the plaque to platelets and coagulation factors in the blood. Such lesions need not be stenotic prior to the acute presentation, which explains why many ACS events are unheralded. The nature of the occlusion (partial or total; transient, intermittent or fixed) and location (proximal or distal and the specific coronary artery affected) largely determine the clinical presentation and course.

Risk Factors for Coronary Atherothrombosis

- Prior ACS
- Tobacco smoking
- Family history
- Diabetes mellitus
- Hypertension
- Elevated low density lipoprotein-cholesterol (LDL)
- Low level of high density lipoprotein-cholesterol (HDL)

Additional risk factors

- Elevated markers of inflammation, including C-reactive protein, interleukin-6 and tumor necrosis factor
- Obesity
- Sedentary lifestyle

Table 6.1 Classification of Acute Coronary Syndromes

	Troponin	EKG
STEMI	Normal or elevated	• ST elevation • Left bundle branch block
Non-STEMI	Normal or elevated	• Normal • Abnormal, but unchanged ST segment depression • T wave inversion
Unstable angina	Normal	

- High apolipoprotein B
- Low apolipoprotein AI
- High lipoprotein (a)
- High plasma homocysteine

Non-atherosclerotic Causes of Acute MI

These warrant consideration in specific patients but are less common.
- Embolus, e.g. vegetation in infective endocarditis
- Spontaneous coronary dissection
- Intense spasm, e.g. in cocaine abuse
- Coronary arteritis (e.g. Kawasaki disease)
- Thrombosis in situ in pro-coaguable states
- Trauma—avulsed coronary artery
- Aortic dissection
- Iatrogenic due to coronary intervention

Acute ST Elevation Myocardial Infarction

This is a medical emergency usually caused by thrombotic occlusion of a major epicardial coronary artery. Irreversible ischemic injury to the myocardium is threatened (or may have occurred at presentation). Prompt action conserves myocardium and prevents complications, including death.

Pathology

MI mostly affects the left ventricle. It usually results from sudden occlusion of a coronary artery or one of its branches by thrombosis over a pre-existing atheromatous plaque. Patients with IHD are at risk of sustaining an MI if additional stresses are placed upon their already critically impaired myocardial circulation.

History

The classic presentation is of sudden onset, severe, constant central chest discomfort, which radiates to the arms, neck, or jaw. The pain is described as a pressure or crushing sensation, similar in nature to previous angina pectoris, but is much more severe and often unrelieved by NTG. The pain is usually accompanied by one or more associated symptoms of sweating, nausea, vomiting, and shortness of breath.

Atypical presentation is relatively common, so adopt a high level of suspicion in order not to miss it. Many patients describe atypical pain, some attributing it to indigestion (be wary of new onset dyspeptic pain in adulthood). Up to a third of patients with acute MI do not report any chest pain. These patients tend to be older, more likely to be female, have a history of diabetes or heart failure, and have a higher mortality. These patients may present with:

- LVF
- Collapse or syncope (often with associated injuries)
- Confusion
- Stroke
- An incidental EKG finding at a later date

In a patient who presents with possible MI, remember to enquire about past medical history (IHD, hypertension, diabetes, hyperlipidemia) and contraindications to thrombolysis (see below). Ask about a drug history, including drugs of abuse (particularly cocaine).

Physical Exam

As with other potentially life-threatening emergencies, examination and initial resuscitation (O_2, IV access, analgesia) go hand in hand. The patient may be pale, sweaty, and distressed. Specific physical signs are absent unless complications have supervened (such as arrhythmias or LVF). Direct your initial examination towards searching for these complications and excluding alternative diagnoses:

- Check pulse, BP, and monitor trace (look for arrhythmia or cardiogenic shock)
- Listen to the heart (are there murmurs or a 3rd heart sound?)
- Listen to the lung fields (is there evidence of LVF, pneumonia, or a pneumothorax?)
- Check that peripheral pulses are present in all limbs (is this aortic dissection?)
- Check the legs for evidence of DVT (is this a PE?)
- Palpate for abdominal tenderness or masses (is this an abdominal emergency such as cholecystitis, pancreatitis, a perforated peptic ulcer, or a ruptured abdominal aortic aneurysm?)

Investigation

The diagnosis of acute MI requires two out of the following three features:

- A history of cardiac-type ischemic chest discomfort
- Evolutionary changes on serial EKGs
- A rise and fall in serum cardiac markers

Note that 50–60% of patients may not have a diagnostic EKG on arrival and up to 17% will have an entirely normal initial EKG. Late presentation does not improve diagnostic accuracy of the EKG. The ED investigation should consist of the following:

- The diagnosis of MI within the first few hours is based upon history and EKG changes. Serum cardiac enzymes may take several hours to rise (see below).
- Record the EKG as soon as possible, ideally within the first few minutes of arrival at hospital. Sometimes patients arrive at hospital with EKGs of diagnostic quality already recorded by paramedics. If the initial EKG is normal, but symptoms suspicious, repeat the EKG every 20–30 minutes and re-evaluate patient clinically.
- Request or download the old records (these may contain previous EKGs for comparison).
- Ensure continuous cardiac monitoring and pulse oximetry.
- Monitor BP and respiratory rate.
- Get venous access and send blood for cardiac enzymes, CMP, and CBC.
- Arterial blood gases are not indicated as they rarely influence treatment and may result in bleeding during thrombolysis.

Cardiac Enzymes

Creatine kinase (CK), aspartate transaminase (AST), and lactate dehydrogenase rise and fall in a recognized sequence following an acute MI. The aminotransferases have been largely replaced by enzymes more specific to cardiac cells, namely the MB subform of creatinine kinase (CK-MB), myoglobin, and cardiac troponin. None of these can be used to exclude an acute MI in the setting of the ED; do not discharge a patient on the basis of a single normal blood test. CK-MB has a higher cardiac specificity than CK. CK-MB is 78–100% sensitive for acute MI at 6 hours after the onset of pain.

These tests may be employed as part of a strategy to rule out MI, but only after a minimum of 6 hours observation with serial EKGs and cardiac enzymes. Troponin T (cTnT) and Troponin I (cTnI) are proteins virtually exclusive to cardiac myocytes. They are highly specific and sensitive, but are only maximally accurate after 12 hours. Therefore, Troponin T and I cannot be used to rule out MI in the first few hours of chest pain.

Thus it is vital that you recognize that the diagnosis of acute coronary syndrome is in the first instance clinical—the initial management is based on clinical diagnosis and the EKG(s) and is not contingent on the troponin result. The troponin may turn out to be elevated and in NSTEMI patients is one of the markers of increased risk (p. 58) but importantly, may be normal in patients with unstable angina who are at high risk of subsequent cardiac events, and the clinical diagnosis is crucial in these patients.

Furthermore, release of troponin T is not specific to coronary disease. Caution is necessary in interpreting an elevated serum troponin in the absence of a typical history and/or ECG changes, particularly where the rise is relatively modest. Other conditions that can lead to troponin elevation include:

- Myocarditis
- Pericarditis
- Pulmonary embolism
- Sepsis
- Renal failure

Radiological Studies

Obtain a CXR only if there is clinical evidence of LVF and if it will not delay thrombolysis (but bear in mind that many medical admission teams will require a routine CXR). It is useful as a screening tool to exclude aortic dissection. Patients with evidence of cardiogenic shock require an urgent bedside ED ECHO (see p. 22).

Immediate Intervention

There are two interventions for acute MI that you offer in the ED. The first is stabilizing or supportive therapies, and the second is initiating reperfusion therapies.

- Speed is of the essence—time really is muscle. Work efficiently as a team to ensure treatment is not delayed.
- If it has not already been administered, give 0.4 mg NTG SL (beware of hypotension—if this occurs, lay the patient flat). Repeat up to three doses separated by 5 minute intervals.
- Provide increments of IV opioid analgesia titrated to effect (e.g. 4 mg morphine IV every 5–10 minutes).
- Give an antiemetic (e.g. 10 mg metoclopramide IV).
- Give 300 mg aspirin PO, unless already given or contraindicated (allergy, active peptic ulcer).
- Check for contraindications to thrombolysis (see below), explain the procedure and possible risks and ensure the patient understands and assents.
- Administer thrombolysis and monitor carefully for hypotension or arrhythmias. Make sure that there is a defibrillator close at

hand. Aim to give thrombolysis within 15 minutes of the patient's arrival at hospital. Start LMWH (e.g. enoxaparin 1 mg/kg IV stat) or heparin according to local protocols.

- If the pain continues, start IV NTG (start at 0.6 mg/h and increase as necessary), provided the systolic BP is above 90 mmHg.
- Beta blockers should be given unless the pulse is less than 60 beats per minute or the BP is less than 100 mmHg. Give metoprolol (5 mg IV every 5 minutes ×3 doses).

Consultation

Make certain that you are following your local protocol when you initiate therapy. Most protocols will call for an early cardiology consultation, and this will certainly be required if you are at a center that performs emergent PTCA. The cardiology team (whether interventional or not) should be paged to the ED simultaneously with your making the diagnosis. Once the patient has been stabilized, contact the PCP and inform her of the situation.

Disposition and Documentation

All patients with evidence of acute infarction are admitted to the ICU. The following key points need to be documented:

- Administration of aspirin
- Administration of β-blockers
- Administration of nitrates (IV, PO, or to the chest wall)
- Administration of analgesia
- Administration of heparin or LMWH and glycoprotein IIb/IIIa inhibitors according to your ED policy or cardiology request
- Time of call to cardiology fellow or attending
- Verify placement of two IV lines
- Time and content of discussion with PCP.

Chest Pain Assessment Units

These units are becoming established in many EDs. A combination of EKGs, ST segment monitoring, cardiac enzymes and exercise testing is used to allow discharge of low to moderate risk patients within 6–12 hours. Remember that simply excluding an acute coronary syndrome is only part of the assessment of chest pain.

Coronary Artery Anatomy

The **left anterior descending** (LAD) coronary artery runs in the anterior interventricular groove supplying the *anterior wall* of the heart. It gives off **septal** branches that supply blood to the *anterior 2/3 of the interventricular septum*, including the *left bundle branch*, **diagonal** vessels to the *lateral wall* of the left ventricle and has a terminal bifurcation that supplies the *apex* of the left ventricle and sometimes wraps around to supply the *inferior wall* of the left ventricle.

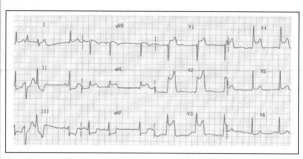

Figure 6.1 ECG in acute anterolateral MI.
There is marked ST segment elevation in leads V1–V4 and aVL. Reciprocal ST segment depression is present in leads II, III and aVF.

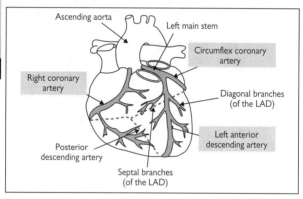

Figure 6.2 There are three principal coronary arteries. The left main stem arises from the left aortic sinus and soon gives rise to the (1) left anterior descending and (2) circumflex coronary arteries. The (3) right coronary artery has a separate origin in the right aortic sinus.

The **circumflex** (LCX) artery runs posteriorly in the left atrio-ventricular groove, giving **obtuse marginal** branches to the *lateral wall* of the left ventricle and supplying the *posterior wall* of the left ventricle.

The **right** coronary artery (RCA) runs in the right atrioventricular groove. It gives branches to the *sino atrial node*, *atrioventricular node,* and *right ventricle*. On reaching the posterior interventricular groove, it gives rise to the **posterior descending artery** that supplies the *inferior wall* of the left ventricle, and the *inferior 1/3 of the interventricular septum*. This is the more common variant. However, in about 10% of patients, the circumflex gives rise to the posterior descending artery and is then termed 'dominant.'

Table 6.2 Coronary Artery Anatomy		
Site of Arterial Occlusion	Myocardial Territory	EKG Changes
LAD	Antero-lateral Antero-septal	V_4–V_6; I, VL V_1–V_4 LBBB
LCX	Posterior	Mirror image changes in V_1–V_2 or V_3 i.e. ST segment depression ± inferior changes; tall R in V_1 May be electrically silent on standard 12-lead ECG
RCA	Inferior wall of LV Right ventricle	II, III, aVF ST elevation V_4R to V_6R

Reperfusion Therapy

Make sure that you are familiar with the acute MI protocol of your institution. Most hospitals have multi-disciplinary teams to accelerate provision of reperfusion therapy. The goals are prompt restoration of coronary flow and myocardial perfusion. Delays increase myocardial necrosis, decrease the efficacy of eventual reperfusion therapy and increase mortality. Reperfusion therapy with thrombolysis or with percutaneous coronary intervention (PCI) is acceptable. Rapid action is vital: The door-to-needle time (thrombolysis) should be <20 minutes and the door-to-balloon time (for primary PCI) should be <60 minutes.

Primary Percutaneous Coronary Intervention

Primary PCI refers to immediate PCI as the initial reperfusion strategy. It achieves high levels of vessel patency and, in experienced hands, may reduce mortality compared to thrombolysis. The risk of stroke is also lower compared to thrombolysis.

- Initiate immediate management measures (see above).
- Alert the cardiac catheterization laboratory at the earliest opportunity.
- In discussion with the interventional cardiologist, it is reasonable to start the glycoprotein IIb/IIIa receptor inhibitor abciximab once the decision for primary PCI has been made.
- Informed consent will be obtained by the interventional team.
- If there is likely to be more than minor delay (i.e., >60 minutes door-to-balloon) before PCI, thrombolysis may be more appropriate, particularly if the symptom duration is less than 3 hours.

Reperfusion Therapy—Angioplasty versus Thrombolysis

Percutaneous transluminal coronary angioplasty (PTCA) is more effective than thrombolysis, and is now the therapy of choice in centers where it is available. Once the diagnosis of an acute MI is made, you should immediately call for the interventional cardiologist. However, PTCA is not universally available, and if you are in a community setting without interventional cardiology, you will need to decide between initiating thrombolysis and transferring the patient to a tertiary center. This will require you deciding whether angioplasty performed after a patient is transferred to a facility where it is available is superior to thrombolytic therapy administered at your (referral) hospital. There is some evidence that the strategy of transfer may improve outcomes, especially if the transfer takes less than two hours, but there is plenty of debate. If you face this dilemma, discuss the options with both the patient (and family) and the consulting cardiologist.

Thrombolysis

Thrombolysis can reperfuse infarcting myocardium and dramatically reverse ST changes. It significantly improves outcomes and should be given as soon as possible, unless your local protocol calls for angioplasty rather than thrombolysis. Ensure that the patient is involved in any decision to thrombolyse.

Indications for Thrombolysis

- ST elevation of >1 mm in 2 limb leads, or
- ST elevation of ≥2 mm in 2 or more contiguous chest leads, or
- LBBB in the presence of a typical history of acute MI (note that the LBBB does not have to be new).

Contraindications to Thrombolysis

Most contraindications are only relative, but they need to be discussed with the patient. In cases of doubt, consult with cardiology before starting thrombolysis. Patients with contraindications to thrombolysis should undergo primary PCI.

Absolute[1]

- Any prior intracranial hemorrhage
- Known intracranial structural vascular lesions (e.g. arteriovenous malformation)
- Known intracranial malignant neoplasm (primary or secondary)
- Ischemic stroke within 3 months
- Active bleeding or bleeding diathesis
- Significant head trauma within 3 months.

Relative[1]

- Severe hypertension (systolic >180 mmHg; diastolic >110 mmHg) despite treatment

[1] Modified from Antman EM, Anbe DT, Armstrong PW, et al. (2004). ACC/AHA guidelines for the management of patients with ST elevation myocardial infarction. *Circulation* 110, 588–636.

- Traumatic or prolonged CPR
- Major surgery within 3 weeks
- Non-compressible vascular punctures
- Recent (within 2–4 weeks) internal bleeding
- Pregnancy
- Active peptic ulcer
- Current anticoagulant use
- Pain for >24 hours
- For streptokinase: prior exposure to streptokinase (persistent antibodies).

Choice of Thrombolytic Agents

Both streptokinase and alteplase (rt-PA) reduce mortality. Alteplase results in about 10 fewer deaths per 1000 patients treated, at the expense of 3 additional strokes compared to streptokinase. Angiographic patency and flow at 90 minutes in the infarct-related artery are directly related to 30-day mortality.

Streptokinase is a traditional thrombolytic agent. However, it is probably inferior to tPA in patients older than 75 with an anterior MI, or an anterior MI in patients under 75 years old within 4 hours of the onset of symptoms, or hypotensive (systolic BP<90 mmHg) patients. Give 1.5 million units by continuous IV infusion over 1 hour. Streptokinase is allergenic. If allergic symptoms develop, give chlorphenamine (10 mg IV) and hydrocortisone (100 mg IV). It also frequently causes hypotension. If this occurs, increase the IV infusion rate and tilt the head of the bed down; treatment rarely needs to be discontinued.

Alteplase (recombinant tissue plasminogen activator—rtPA) is non-allergenic and non-antigenic. It is most effective given by the accelerated regimen: 15 mg IV bolus, followed by 0.75 mg/kg (up to 50 mg) IV for 30 minutes, then 0.5 mg/kg (up to 35 mg) IV over 60 minutes. In addition, give LMWH (e.g. enoxaparin 1 mg/kg IV) or heparin concomitantly through a separate IV line (5000 units IV bolus, then 1000 units/h IV), according to your local protocol.

Reteplase (modified tPA) has a longer half life than standard tPA, and may reduce the time to perfusion. It is given as two IV boluses of 10 units separated by 30 minutes apart. In addition, give LMWH or heparin as for tPA.

Reperfusion is suggested by resolution of ST segment elevation by >50% following thrombolysis and relief of pain.

Failure to reperfuse

Failure of symptoms and/or ST segment elevation to resolve by >50% 60–90 minutes after thrombolysis may result from a failure to achieve patency of the epicardial vessel or due to distal (microvascular) occlusion. The optimal course of action is uncertain. There is no clear benefit from repeat thrombolysis or from 'salvage/rescue' PCI.

Trials to resolve this uncertainty are ongoing. Salvage PCI is usually recommended in the presence of ongoing symptoms or electrical or hemodynamic instability.

Additional Treatments

- An ACE inhibitor, e.g. ramipril 2.5 mg qd or lisinopril 5 mg qd, should be commenced within the first 24 hours following acute MI if the systolic blood pressure is >100 mmHg. There is particular benefit in the presence of left ventricular dysfunction. The dose should be titrated upwards as blood pressure permits
- Statin treatment should be instigated in almost all patients
- The anti-platelet agent clopidogrel administered at presentation and continued at a dose of 75 mg daily for 4 weeks, in addition to standard therapy, reduces the 30-day risk of a composite of death, re-infarction, and stroke inpatients undergoing non-invasive management
- In post-STEMI patients with left ventricular ejection fraction <40%, already receiving an ACE inhibitor and with either symptomatic heart failure or diabetes, but without significant renal dysfunction or hyperkalemia, there is a benefit from aldosterone blockade
- Diabetic patients should receive an insulin infusion based on a sliding scale.

Risk Stratification and Prognosis

An important predictor of 30-day mortality in acute MI is the presence (and degree) of heart failure, quantified by Killip in 1967 and updated from GUSTO trial data for the thrombolytic era (Table 6.3 below).

Table 6.3 Acute MI, Prognostic Indicators		
Group	Clinical Feature	30-day Mortality (%)
Killip class I	No S3 and clear lungs	5.1
Killip class II	S3 or crepitations in lungs	13.6
Killip class III	Crepitations >50% of lung	32.2
Killip class IV	Shock	57.8
Anterior MI		9.9
Inferior MI		5.0
Age <60 years		2.4
Age 60–75 years		7.9
Age >75 years		20.5

Reprinted with permission from Lee KL, Woodlief LH, Topol E J, et al. Predictors of 30-day mortality in the era of reperfusion for acute myocardial infarction. *Circulation* 1996; 91: 1659–1668.

Differential Diagnosis

- Anxiety
- Aortic dissection
- Biliary colic
- Costochondritis
- Esophagitis
- Herpes zoster

- Myocardial ischemia
- Peptic ulcer disease
- Pericarditis
- Pneumonia
- Pneumothorax
- Pulmonary embolism

Complications of Acute MI

Immediate Complications (Within Hours)

Arrhythmias

These occur in over 75% of patients with an acute MI. The most common rhythms seen are sinus tachycardia, and atrial or ventricular premature beats. Transient AF occurs in about 15% and requires no treatment. Watch for sudden VT/VF and treat as on p. 274.

Complete heart block

Usually occurring in the context of acute inferior MI, CHB is often transient, resolving with reperfusion. Where hemodynamic compromise occurs, insertion of a temporary transvenous pacing wire may be indicated. Resolution of CHB may take several days, so be patient before prescribing a permanent pacemaker. Complete heart block in the context of anterior MI suggests extensive infarction, and adverse prognosis. Temporary pacing should be considered (p. 251).

Hypotension

Hypotension in the absence of signs of heart failure may respond to a fluid challenge, e.g. 250–500 mL normal saline given rapidly. Acute inferior MI is often accompanied by right ventricular infarction.

Right ventricular infarction

This occurs in about 30% of inferior MI, and is suggested by ST elevation >1 mm in V_4R. It carries an adverse prognosis. Hypotension is common which may require robust fluid resuscitation to maintain left-sided filling pressures.

Hypokalemia

Treat if the potassium is below 4 mmol/L (e.g. 20 mmol KCl in 100 mL 0.9% saline IV over 1 hour), together with magnesium (5 mL 50% in 100 mL 0.9% saline IV over 1 hour).

Cardiogenic shock (see p. 22).

Cardiogenic shock is defined as poor cardiac output with evidence of tissue hypoxia which does not improve with correction of intravascular volume. The mortality is 50–80%. The evaluation and treatment is detailed on p. 27. Echocardiography may be required to exclude

53

conditions requiring urgent surgical repair (e.g. mitral regurgitation from papillary muscle rupture, aortic dissection, ventricular septum rupture, cardiac tamponade from ventricular wall rupture). Once these are excluded start inotropic support (p. 28) and/or intra-aortic balloon counter pulsation (p. 32). Within 36 hours of acute MI, emergency PCI should be considered.

Pulmonary congestion and pulmonary edema

Give oxygen, morphine, and intravenous loop diuretics, e.g. furosemide 40–100 mg IV. Infuse NTG 0.5–10 mg/h IV if BP >90 mmHg systolic. Obtain a CXR. Insert a urinary catheter and monitor urine output hourly. Give oxygen and monitor the O_2 saturation with pulse oximetry. In severe cases, CPAP or intubation and ventilation may be required (p. 30). Keep the patient's relatives informed.

Early Complications (Within Days)

Reinfarction

Surprisingly, the optimal course of action in reinfarction following initially successful reperfusion is uncertain. Many would proceed to angiography and PCI (or coronary artery bypass) in the presence of ongoing symptoms or electrical or hemodynamic instability. It is reasonable to re-administer thrombolysis in patients for whom PCI is not available within 60 minutes (but remember that streptokinase should not be given more than once).

New murmur

A new murmur and abrupt hemodynamic deterioration suggest the possibility of papillary muscle rupture (or dysfunction), ventricular septal defect or free wall rupture. Obtain a stat echocardiogram and page the cardiothoracic surgeon. In general, a structural problem needs a structural fix.

Mitral regurgitation (MR)

Acute severe MR due to papillary muscle rupture is a cardiac surgical emergency. Stabilization can be attempted with intravenous diuretics, intravenous nitrates, and intra-aortic balloon counterpulsation (p. 32) but these are temporizing measures at best. Urgent surgical repair should be performed.

Ventricular septal rupture

Acquired VSD requires urgent surgical repair. Stabilization can be attempted with intravenous diuretics, intravenous nitrates, and intra-aortic balloon pump insertion (p. 32).

Rupture of myocardial free wall

Abrupt deterioration within 3 days post MI may indicate myocardial rupture. If not fatal, urgent surgical repair will be needed.

Pericarditis

Pericarditis is common after myocardial infarction. The pain is usually pleuritic, positional, and distinct from the ischemia-related pain of the initial presentation. Pericarditis occurs >12 hours after acute MI and is treated with high dose non-steroidals. Anticoagulation should be stopped if a pericardial effusion develops or enlarges.

Mural thrombus and systemic embolization

Full anti-coagulation with heparin (and subsequently warfarin) should be obtained in patients with large anterior MI, known LV thrombus, or atrial fibrillation, all of which are associated with an increased risk of systemic embolization. Aspirin should usually be continued.

Late Complications (Several Weeks)

Dressler syndrome

This is an auto-immune mediated acute febrile illness that occurs 2 weeks to several months after acute MI. The incidence has fallen in the reperfusion era. Management is with aspirin or NSAIDs. Large pericardial effusions may accumulate causing hemodynamic embarrassment or even tamponade. Obtain an echocardiogram. Stop anti-coagulants to minimize the risk of hemorrhagic transformation. Percutaneous drainage may be required (p. 254).

Ventricular tachycardia

Scar formation post myocardial infarction predisposes to ventricular tachycardia (p. 100). In selected patients implantable cardioverter-defibrillator (ICD) therapy is indicated.

Left ventricular aneurysm

Infarcted tissue may become thinned and dyskinetic. Aneurysms are hemodynamically inefficient, predispose to thrombus formation, and may cause persistent ST elevation on the EKG. Depending on their size and location, they may require long term anticoagulation. They strongly predispose to ventricular arrhythmias, and an EP evaluation is warranted. In some cases they can be resected surgically.

Post Infarct Management

In the absence of complications or persistent ischemia, patients should be mobile within 24 hours. At day 3–5 a pre-discharge sub-maximal exercise test may be undertaken. A low-level positive test indicates further myocardium at risk, and pre-discharge angiography is usually indicated. A negative test indicates a low-risk group and is helpful to rebuild patient confidence.

Take the opportunity to implement education on secondary prevention, e.g. smoking cessation and diet (low saturated fat, low salt, promote Mediterranean-type diet). Introduction to a supervised, structured rehabilitation program is generally beneficial.

Discharge Medication

- Aspirin
- Beta-blocker
- ACE inhibitor
- Statin
- Clopidogrel

Unstable Angina and Non ST Elevation MI

In the absence of sustained ST segment elevation, ischemic pain of abruptly worsening severity or occurring at rest is classed as 'unstable angina' or non-ST segment elevation MI (NSTEMI). The distinction depends on the eventual presence (NSTEMI) or absence (UA) of an elevated troponin measurement. The underlying pathology (ruptured or eroded coronary plaque with non-occlusive or intermittently occlusive thrombus) and initial management are the same. The immediate objectives are to relieve pain and to prevent progression to acute MI.

Symptoms

Central chest pain of various severity and duration, possibly radiating to the jaw or (left) arm and typically not relieved by nitrates. Pain is sometimes accompanied by diaphoresis, nausea, and vomiting. There may be a history of prior chronic stable angina.

Signs

Pain or distress and clammy skin (a result of sweating and cutaneous vasoconstriction). Occasionally accompanied by intermittent pulmonary edema, depending on degree of ischemia and underlying left ventricular function. There may be no abnormal physical signs.

Investigations

Remember that the initial diagnosis is clinical.

- The EKG may be normal
- EKG changes include ST segment depression and T wave inversion, which may be 'dynamic,' that is, coming and going with symptoms
- Exclude sustained ST segment elevation (p. 43)
- If the EKG is normal but pain persists, obtain serial EKGs
- Check the CBC to exclude anemia
- Obtain a troponin at presentation and at 6 and 12 hours after the onset of pain.

Immediate Management

- Oxygen
- Aspirin 150–300 mg chewed to achieve rapid buccal absorption

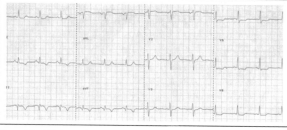

Figure 6.3 EKG during chest pain.
ST segment depression in leads I, V5 and V6 with T wave inversion in leads II, III and aVF is suggestive of ischemia in the inferolateral territory.

- Clopidogrel 300 mg po then 75 mg daily
- Low molecular weight heparin
- Sublingual or intravenous nitrates
- Morphine 5–10 mg IV for analgesia and anxiety
- Metoclopramide 10 mg IV
- Beta-blocker, e.g. atenolol 50 mg po or metoprolol 25–50 mg
- Oral diltiazem is an alternative when beta-blockers are contraindicated (and there is no evidence of cardiac failure, atrioventricular block, or hypotension)
- Revascularization in selected patients according to risk.

Glycoprotein IIb/IIIa Inhibition

Glycoprotein IIb/IIIa inhibitors are potent anti-platelet agents that block the common path of platelet aggregation. Patients undergoing PCI may benefit from administration of abciximab prior to the procedure, while patients with high risk features (see below) or evidence of ongoing pain or ischemia may benefit from eptifibatide or tirofiban (but not abciximab) even where early PCI is not planned.

Risk Stratification and Early Invasive Treatment

Evidence from randomized trials suggests that higher risk patients derive greatest benefit from a strategy of early coronary angiography and revascularization (PCI/coronary artery bypass).

Clinical indications for early invasive strategy include ongoing symptomatic ischemia (especially dynamic ST segment depression on the ECG), hemodynamic compromise, and recent (e.g. within 6 months) PCI. Elevated troponin also suggests a high risk category. The TIMI score is a well-validated, simple risk calculator (see Box 6.1). As a guide, patients with TIMI score >3 are at high risk and early invasive management may be beneficial.

Box 6.1 TIMI Risk Score for Unstable Angina/NSTEMI (1 point for each)

- Age ≥ 65 years
- ≥3 coronary risk factors
- Use of aspirin within 7 days
- Elevated cardiac markers
- ST segment deviation
- Prior angiographic evidence of coronary disease
- More than 2 angina events within 24 hours

The score is determined by simply summing the number of risk factors above. For patients with TIMI score 0–1, the combined risk of death, (re)infarction or recurrent severe ischemia requiring revascularization is about 5% while TIMI score 6–7 confers a risk of 41%.

Recent Percutaneous Coronary Intervention

Insertion of a metallic stent during PCI poses a risk of acute and subacute stent thrombosis. To counter this, the anti-platelet agents aspirin and clopidogrel should be given prior to PCI. Heparin (± abciximab) is given in the cardiac catheterization laboratory. The risk of stent thrombosis declines rapidly during first 24 hours after PCI. For conventional bare metal stents, it is usual to continue a combination of aspirin 75 mg od and clopidogrel 75 mg od for at least one month after PCI to cover the small risk of subacute stent occlusion. Where drug-eluting stents are used, there is a possibility of delayed stent endothelialization and aspirin/clopidogrel combination is usually maintained for 6 months.

Be aware of the possibility of stent-related thrombosis, particularly early after implantation, where drug compliance is questionable or where anti-platelet agents have recently been stopped. Early angiography is indicated.

Chapter 7

Acute Heart Failure

Introduction

Acute heart failure can be either acute or acute-on-chronic (more common). In all cases, efforts should be made to identify the underlying cause, and in particular, why it should present now. Remember that heart failure is not a homogeneous condition and although some general principles apply, successful treatment depends upon the accurate assessment of the etiology and hemodynamic profile in each patient.

Clinical Features

The clinical features are of fluid overload and low cardiac output:

Fluid overload/congestion
- Orthopnea
- Raised JVP*
- Gallop rhythm
- Pulmonary inspiratory crackles
- Peripheral edema*
- Ascites*
- Hepatic distension*

Low output
- Tachycardia
- Low blood pressure/narrow pulse pressure*
- Cool extremities
- Poor capillary refill
- Confusion/drowsiness
- Oliguria
- Pulsus alternans (terminal)

*May be absent in acute heart failure.

If patient is in shock (i.e., a systolic BP <90 mmHg with signs of reduced major organ perfusion), they need urgent intervention, as outlined on p. 22).

Systolic vs. Diastolic Heart Failure

Systolic heart failure is characterized by reduced systolic function on echocardiography or other imaging modality. Diastolic heart failure is characterized by abnormalities of left ventricular filling in the absence of major systolic dysfunction. Diastolic failure is mainly due to increased stiffness of the ventricle, commonly from longstanding hypertension. These patients respond to vasodilators, adequate fluid balance, and rate slowing (if tachycardic); they respond poorly to dehydration. Diastolic heart failure is particularly common in the elderly.

Causes of Decompensation

Many cases of acute heart failure are in fact a worsening or decompensation of chronic heart failure. It is therefore vital to seek the reason for the decompensation. Remember that poor compliance with therapy (either drugs or fluid intake) is a common cause. Other causes are:

- Administration of inappropriate medications (e.g. NSAIDs, antiarrhythmic agents, non-dihydropyridine calcium antagonists)
- Alcohol abuse
- Aortic dissection
- Arrhythmias
- Cardiomyopathy
- Endocrine disorders (thyrotoxicosis)
- Fluid overload (consider renal failure, and iatrogenic causes if in hospital)
- High output failure (consider anemia, hyperthyroidism, and an a-v fistula)
- Hypertension
- Inadequate therapy
- Lack of compliance
- Myocardial ischemia or infarction
- Myocarditis
- Pericardial tamponade
- Pulmonary infection
- Uncontrolled hypertension
- Valvular heart disease

Investigation

- CBC (look for anemia and signs of infection)
- Electrolytes
- Troponin (acute coronary syndrome)
- Thyroid function
- EKG (ischemia, MI)
- Brain natriuretic peptide (BNP)—see below
- Echocardiography

Brain Natriuretic Peptide (BNP)

Many physicians rely on a serum BNP to confirm the diagnosis of acute heart failure. In reality this test is not likely to help in most cases, where it is clinically obvious that the patient has, or does not have, acute CHF. However, in a minority of cases the BNP may help determine the diagnosis. A negative test result makes the diagnosis of heart failure unlikely. Threshold values of >300 pg/mL for NT-proBNP and 100 pg/mL for BNP are used most commonly.

The following may give rise to an elevated BNP in the absence of clinical heart failure:

- Renal failure
- Acute coronary syndromes
- Aortic stenosis

- Mitral regurgitation
- Hypertrophic cardiomyopathy.

Differential Diagnosis

Any cause of shortness of breath (p. 9) may be included here, but the most common causes, particularly without radiographic evidence of pulmonary edema are:

- Chronic obstructive pulmonary disease
- Pulmonary embolus (major pulmonary embolism can however cause pulmonary edema).

Echocardiography is the most useful diagnostic tool for discrimination and may be supplemented by BNP measurement (see above).

For patients presenting with radiological evidence of pulmonary edema, non-cardiogenic causes have to be considered (see Box 7.1). Clinical features suggestive of a non-cardiogenic cause are normal/low venous pressure, normal/increased cardiac output, normal EKG, normal LV function on Echo, and a failure to respond to standard heart failure therapy.

Box 7.1 Causes of Non-cardiogenic Pulmonary Edema

- Imbalance of Starling's forces
- Increased pulmonary capillary pressure
- Decreased plasma oncotic pressure (hypoalbuminemia)
- Decreased interstitial pressure (decompression of pneumothorax, severe asthma)
- Increased alveolar-capillary permeability (ARDS)
- Infection
- Toxins
- Aspiration of gastric contents
- Disseminated intravascular coagulation (DIC)
- Acute pancreatitis
- Drugs
- 'Shock-lung'
- Other
  - Lymphatic insufficiency
  - High altitude
  - Pulmonary embolism
  - Neurogenic
  - Eclampsia
  - Post CABG/cardioversion
  - Post anesthesia.

Management

Immediate Management

The immediate treatment aims are to reduce both preload and after-load with a combination of diuretics and vasodilators. In addition, it is vital to insure adequate oxygenation; this has a major impact on myocardial performance and the response to diuretic therapy. Initial steps are

- Oxygen therapy
- Morphine 2–6 mg IV, repeat as needed every 10–15 minutes
- Loop diuretics (e.g. furosemide 40–120 mg IV)
- IV nitrates (e.g. NTG 1–10 mg/h) are useful if significant failure but be sure the systolic blood pressure is adequate (i.e. >95 mmHg)
- Withdraw any drugs which may be contributing to heart failure (e.g. calcium channel blockers and NSAIDs).

Continuing Management

Drug therapy can be tailored according to the hemodynamic profile and fluid overload (see opposite).

ACE inhibitors

- Not usually introduced in the acute phase of heart failure although there is evidence for their early introduction in patients following MI
- In the long term they are beneficial, including a reduction in mortality

They should be withdrawn temporarily in the following circumstances:

- Systolic BP <80 mmHg or <100 mmHg in the presence of renal impairment or diuretic resistance
- Creatinine >300 mmol/L
- Progressive rise in creatinine of >25–30%
- They can be introduced/reintroduced when fluid status is optimal and the patient is hemodynamically stable.

Beta-blockers

- Contraindicated in acute heart failure
- In all but mild cases with predominant fluid overload, they should be withdrawn temporarily
- Can be (re)introduced when the patient has been stabilized, and fluid balance is optimal but this may take several days or even weeks.

Box 7.2 Hemodynamic Profiles in Heart Failure

(warm/cold = peripheral perfusion; wet/dry = congested/not congested)

Warm and wet (common)
- Emphasis on diuretic therapy with addition of vasodilators
- Significant diuresis may be required
- Beta-blockers can be continued
- Inotropes inappropriate.

Cold and wet
- Emphasis on vasodilator therapy with additional diuretics
- Beta-blockers and ACE inhibitors may need temporary withdrawal
- Vasodilating inotropes (e.g. dobutamine) may be helpful if poor response.

Warm and dry
- Target profile
- Emphasis on titration of chronic therapy to optimal doses.

Cold and dry
- → Distinguish from hypovolemic shock
- Emphasis on inotropic support intra-aortic balloon pump
- Hemodynamic monitoring required
- Cautious filling if CXR clear.

Source: Nohria A, Lewis E, Stevenson LW. *JAMA* 2002; 287: 628–640.

Diuretics

Loop
- Standard therapy in acute pulmonary edema and in patients demonstrating signs of fluid overload
- Infusions are more effective than bolus regimens (this is because time above the natriuretic threshold is more important than maximum concentration in the nephron)
- Start with furosemide 40 mg IV if not on diuretics or, if previously treated, with normal oral dose given intravenously and titrate according to the response
- In cases of severe heart failure, diuretic resistance, or renal impairment consider a furosemide bolus followed by an infusion over 4–8 hours. The maximum bolus dose is 100 mg, and the maximum infusion rate is 4 mg/min.

Non-loop
- Thiazides and aldosterone antagonists are useful as an adjunct to loop diuretics in diuretic resistance
- Hydrochlorthiazide 25–50 mg twice daily (ineffective when the creatinine clearance is <30 mL/min)

- Metolazone (2.5–10 mg daily) has an effect regardless of creatinine clearance and produces a more rapid diuresis. Care is required, however, due to its potent effect
- Aldosterone antagonists
- Spironolactone (25–50 mg daily).

Digoxin

- There is no role for digoxin in the management of acute CHF.

Vasodilators

- Morphine is a potent venodilator and anxiolytic. Give 4–6 mg IV and repeat as needed
- Nitrates
- Sub-lingual nitroglycerin is often very helpful, but if the patient has severe CHF give it IV. Start with 5 mcg/min and closely monitor the blood pressure
- Oral may be added, though evidence for usefulness is poor
- Nitrates are venodilators at low doses and arterial vasodilators in high dose

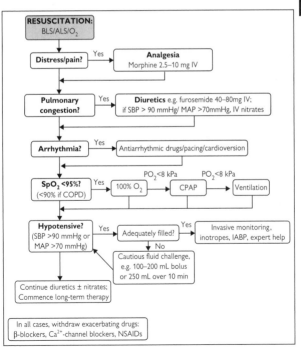

Figure 7.1 Management algorithm for patients presenting with acute heart failure.

- Tolerance occurs after 24 hours
- Aim for a 10 mmHg fall in systolic blood pressure
- Discontinue if blood pressure falls below 90 mmHg.

Sodium nitroprusside (see p. 148)

This should be reserved for severe cases.

- Start at 0.5–5 µg/kg/min IV infusion
- Requires arterial pressure monitoring

Prolonged use is associated with toxicity and should be avoided in patients with severe renal or hepatic failure. It is most useful in hypertensive heart failure and acute mitral regurgitation.

Monitoring and Goals

Monitoring

Pulse, BP, EKG monitoring, pulse oximetry

- Automatically in first 24 hours
- Prolonged in the presence of arrhythmias, during inotrope therapy or in the case of persistent hemodynamic instability.

Arterial blood gases

- These are not very useful, but are often still part of the routine labs obtained on admission of patients with severe heart failure. Check with your colleagues if you are not sure about ordering an ABG.
- Regularly in patients on continuous positive airways pressure (CPAP).

Electrolytes, creatinine and renal function

- Daily in patients who are hemodynamically unstable, and patients on intravenous or combination diuretics.

Fluid balance/urinary catheterization

- Fluid balance is recommended in all cases
- Urinary catheterization used to be routinely done in patients with severe heart failure. However, this routine practice led to avoidable urinary tract infections, which are bad for the patient (and are no-longer reimbursed by Medicare). Urinary catheterization should therefore generally be avoided and performed on a case-by-case basis.

CVP (see p. 31)

This is not usually required. It is difficult to perform insertion in a patient with pulmonary edema, but may guide therapy when inotropic support is needed.

Pulmonary artery catheter

This, too, is rarely required, but is useful to exclude non-cardiogenic pulmonary edema. The measurements may be misleading in mitral stenosis, aortic regurgitation, high airway pressures, and poor LV compliance.

Goals of Therapy

Without hemodynamic monitoring

- Symptomatic improvement
- Oxygenation SaO_2 >95%
- Warm peripheries
- Systolic BP >90 mmHg
- JVP (isolated right heart failure excluded) <5 cm
- Clinical and radiological resolution of pulmonary edema
- Urine output >0.5 mL/kg/h.

With hemodynamic monitoring (as above plus)

- Pulmonary wedge pressure 16–18 mmHg
- Cardiac output >2.5 L/min/m^2
- Systemic vascular resistance 950–1300 dyne-seconds/cm^2.

Box 7.3 New York Heart Association (NYHA) Classification of Heart Failure

Class I	Asymptomatic (though with reduced LV function). No limitation of physical activity.
Class II	Mildly symptomatic, with slight limitation of physical activity. Comfortable at rest but ordinary physical activity results in fatigue or dyspnea.
Class III	Moderately symptomatic, with marked limitation of physical activity. Comfortable at rest but less than ordinary activity results in fatigue or dyspnea.
Class IV	Severely symptomatic. Unable to carry out any physical activity without discomfort. Includes dyspnea/fatigue at rest, with any activity resulting in increased discomfort.

Source: American Heart Association, Inc.

Special Circumstances

Intractable Pulmonary Edema and Hypoxia

(pO_2 < 60 mmHg, pCO_2 > 50 mmHg, worsening acidosis)

Non-invasive ventilation

Two forms of non-invasive ventilation can be used: CPAP and BiPAP. These may be particularly helpful in patients with reversible ischemia.

BiPAP may, however, increase cardiac work and should be used with caution.

Invasive ventilation

Should be considered in the following circumstances:

- Worsening mental status
- Failure to correct hypoxia (SaO_2 <90%)
- Fatigue associated with acidosis (pH <7.2)
- Failure to tolerate CPAP mask.

Hemofiltration

May occasionally be required in the presence of acute renal failure and volume overload, where the etiology of the acute heart failure is felt to be reversible.

Cardiorenal Syndrome

Patients who are aneuric or oliguric despite loop diuretic therapy may require inotropic support (p. 28) and/or hemofiltration.

Acute MI (p. 49)

Revascularization using thrombolysis or primary/rescue angioplasty with balloon pump support if available.

Acute Ventricular Septal Defect/Mitral Valve Rupture

These predominantly mechanical disorders giving rise to pulmonary edema often respond poorly to conventional therapy. Early surgery with balloon pump support prior to surgery is recommended (see p. 32).

Diabetes

Insulin infusion is recommended in diabetics with acute heart failure.

Thyrotoxicosis

Cautious use of non-selective beta-blockade is recommended (propranolol 0.5 mg IV, or 10 mg orally).

Hypertensive Crisis

This is covered in detail on p. 238.

Severe Bronchoconstriction ('Cardiac Asthma')

This is a profound bronchoconstrictor response to pulmonary edema. If conventional therapy fails there may be a response to IV aminophylline (250 mg IV bolus over 20 minutes). Be cautious since this is associated with an incidence of cardiac arrhythmias.

Right Heart Failure

This is particularly seen in the context of RV infarction (usually accompanying inferior MI) and pulmonary embolism. The diagnosis is suggested by clear lung fields in the context of a raised venous pressure and systemic hypotension. Early echocardiography is recommended, and give repeated fluid boluses (e.g. 500 cc normal saline over 15 minutes and repeated as clinically indicated).

Recurrent Admissions with 'Flash' Pulmonary Edema

These patients may have a relatively normal exercise tolerance between attacks. The following differential diagnoses should be considered:

- Renal artery stenosis
- Reversible ischemia
- Tachyarrhythmias.

Severe Aortic Stenosis (p. 133)

Patients with severe aortic stenosis and heart failure are difficult to treat. Diuretics are the mainstay of therapy as a holding measure. Vasodilators and inotropes are contraindicated. The only truly effective treatment is urgent aortic valve replacement. Although the surgical risk may be high, the prognosis is dismal without this intervention.

Box 7.4 Causes of Right Heart Failure

- RV infarction
- Pulmonary embolic disease
- Tamponade
- Chronic pulmonary disease/hypoxia
- Pulmonary hypertension
- Valvular disease
- Congenital heart disease, e.g. Ebstein's anomaly, Eisenmenger syndrome
- Right ventricular dysplasia

Cardiogenic Shock

This is covered in detail on p. 22. In cases of cardiogenic shock with acute heart failure, the prognosis is particularly poor and recovery is unlikely unless there is a reversible cause.

Cardiogenic Shock is Defined by

- Mean arterial pressure <60 mmHg or systolic BP <90 mmHg
- In the presence of:
  - Satisfactory heart rate (60–95 bpm)
  - Adequate filling pressures
  - On 100% oxygen

- With one of the following:
  - Obtunded
  - Poor peripheral perfusion
  - Low urine output
  - Central venous O_2 saturation <70%
  - Lactic acidosis (>2.0 mmol/L).

Treatment (see cardiovascular collapse p. 27)

This is only appropriate in patients where there is a potentially reversible cause or as a bridge to revascularization or transplantation. Treatment consists of:

- Inotropic support
- Intra-aortic balloon pumping
- Mechanical left ventricular assist devices are available in a few centers, again primarily as a bridge to transplantation.

Myocarditis

Causes

- Viral (characteristically enterovirus infections, e.g. coxsackie)
- Other infective causes: bacteria, fungii, rickettsia, and spirochetes
- Cocaine
- Peripartum cardiomyopathy
- Giant cell myocarditis.

Presentation

Patients have a wide spectrum of presentation, from the acute fulminant form, in which the outcome ranges from death to complete recovery, to a chronic form indistinguishable on presentation from a dilated cardiomyopathy.

Clinical Features

Patients present with fatigue, breathlessness and chest discomfort. There may be a fever and a disproportionate tachycardia. Atrial and ventricular arrhythmias are common.

Investigations

- CXR: heart size may be normal or enlarged
- EKG: ST and T wave abnormalities, may present with regional ST elevation and can be mistaken for acute MI. Look for AV block and conduction defects
- Echocardiography: Look for global or regional wall motion abnormalities

- Viral serology: often sent but rarely useful in guiding therapy
- Troponin: elevated in acute cases
- Myocardial biopsy: again rarely helpful in guiding therapy but may be performed at the time of coronary angiography.

Treatment

- Bed rest, ACE inhibitors, diuretics and inotropes as required
- Arrhythmias are treated as for patients with known LV dysfunction. However, patients display an increased sensitivity to digoxin
- Anticoagulation for severe LV dysfunction or LV thrombus
- Cardiac transplantation is the only therapeutic option.

Cardiomyopathies

Hypertrophic Cardiomyopathy

The identification of patients presenting with hypertrophic cardiomyopathy is important, as vasodilators and inotropes are contraindicated. The most likely emergency presentations are with syncope, arrhythmias, or chest pain. Presentation with LV failure is usually secondary to fast AF.

Symptoms

- Syncope
- Chest pain
- Palpitations
- Breathlessness.

Examination

- Can be normal
- Prominent a wave in JVP
- Bifid pulse and/or apex
- Mid systolic murmur in aortic region
- 4th heart sound
- Pan systolic murmur at apex (if mitral regurgitation).

Investigations

EKG: Prominent Q waves in inferior/anterior leads, left atrial enlargement, giant T wave inversion (apical variant), pre-excitation (see opposite).

ECHO: LVH (>13 mm), systolic anterior movement of mitral valve, mitral regurgitation, outflow tract gradient, diastolic dysfunction.

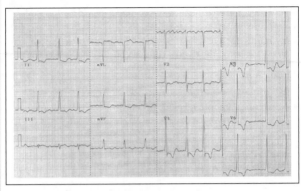

Figure 7.2 EKG in hypertrophic cardiomyopathy.
The underlying rhythm is AF. Tall R waves are seen along with repolarization changes in V3–V6, in keeping with significant LV hypertrophy.

Treatment

- Arrhythmias should be treated according to standard guidelines (see p. 75).
- Digoxin is best avoided and verapamil should be used in patients with an outflow tract gradient
- Emergent cardioversion should be performed for patients in AF who are hypotensive and in pulmonary edema
- Angina can be treated with beta-blockade
- Adequate filling pressures should be maintained, especially in post-operative patients
- In the presence of an outflow tract gradient, inotropes and nitrates are contraindicated, even in the presence of hypotension.

Dilated Cardiomyopathy

This presents with a globally dilated LV and poor function. Treat as for other causes of heart failure. The causes (see below) and reasons for decompensation should be investigated.
Causes:

- Idiopathic (familial)
- Coronary artery disease
- Alcoholic cardiomyopathy
- Hypertension (end-stage)
- Aortic stenosis (end-stage)
- Myocarditis
- Chronic tachyarrhythmia

- Peri-partum cardiomyopathy
- Autoimmune disease
- HIV cardiomyopathy
- Arrhythmogenic right ventricular cardiomyopathy (predominantly RV dilation, but can be LV too)
- Hemochromatosis.

Restrictive Cardiomyopathy

This usually presents as a hypertrophied LV with poor function (especially diastolic function). Like hypertensive heart failure, it requires adequate filling and vasodilators, and minimal diuretics.

Causes:

- Idiopathic
- Myocardial fibrosis (from any cause)
- Amyloidosis
- Sarcoidosis
- Scleroderma
- Iron storage diseases (hemochromatosis, multiple transfusions in thallassemia)
- Diabetic cardiomyopathy
- Eosinophilic heart disease
- Glycogen storage diseases
- Other rare genetic diseases (Fabry's, Hurler's).

Difficult Case Examples

1. AF and Heart Failure

A patient presents in severe pulmonary edema with AF at a rate of 170. Has not responded to 3 doses of furosemide 40 mg IV stat and a loading dose of digoxin. Oxygen saturations are 90% on 100% O_2. Is it safe to cardiovert?

A: Cardioversion under sedation is probably the best option here especially if the patient is hypotensive.

2. Sepsis and Heart Failure

A patient presents with acute dyspnoea and sepsis, a pulse of 110 bpm, a systolic BP 80 mmHg and no visible venous pressure. There is a history of left ventricular failure and the patient does not want to lie flat. What is the appropriate management?

A: Patients with a combination of sepsis and heart failure present difficult management problems. A clear chest X-ray is reassuring and it is then reasonable to institute fluids, but often there is only a portable X-ray which is difficult to interpret. A central line is helpful with a target CVP of 8–10 mmHg. However, it is not advisable to force a patient flat to put in a central line when they are acutely dyspneic: they will be uncomfortable and may become combative. Cautious boluses of 200 cc normal saline can be used but **stay with the patient to monitor the response**. Stop if the patient deteriorates or desaturates. The ICU team should be involved as the patient will require monitoring in that setting.

3. Patient on Beta-blocker Therapy

Q: Patient presents with dyspnea and evidence of left ventricular failure with basal crepitations and an elevated jugular venous pressure. The patient is taking carvedilol 25 mg bid and an ACE inhibitor. Should the beta-blocker be stopped and if so when can it be restarted?

A: If the patient is hemodynamically stable and is not in acute respiratory distress, it is reasonable to continue beta-blocker therapy and increase the diuretic dose. With hemodynamic compromise (hypotension, systolic BP <100 mmHg, or poor perfusion), beta-blocker therapy should be discontinued and restarted when the pulmonary edema has cleared and systolic blood pressure is ≥100 mmHg. The ACE inhibitor should be stopped if there is severe hypotension (systolic BP <80 mmHg) or moderate hypotension (systolic BP 80–100 mmHg) with evidence of deteriorating renal function (oliguria or rising creatinine).

4. Poor Peripheral Perfusion and Pulmonary Edema

Q: A patient presents in pulmonary edema. The patient is cold peripherally, the pulse is 100 bpm (small volume) and the systolic blood pressure is 110 mmHg. The patient has not passed urine for 2 hours despite 100 mg IV lasix. What are the therapeutic options?

A: Patients with evidence of poor tissue perfusion but a reasonable systolic pressure may respond to vasodilating inotropes (e.g. dobutamine or low dose dopamine). Vasodilating inotropes are often started inappropriately late when the systolic blood pressure is low—in this situation they are often ineffective and lower the blood pressure further.

5. Cardiogenic Shock Post-MI

Q: Your patient deteriorated 8 hours after thrombolysis for a large anterior MI. Pulmonary edema and hypotension (systolic blood pressure 80 mmHg) are present. There has been no urine output for 3 hours. What is the appropriate management?

A: This situation carries a very high mortality regardless of any intervention. If there is felt to be a significant reversible component then vasoconstricting inotropes or insertion of an intra-aortic balloon pump is required while awaiting transfer to the catheter laboratory for angioplasty. Advanced support is not indicated if no definitive procedure to restore myocardial function is planned.

Arrhythmias

Bradycardia

Bradycardia is a heart rate of less than 60 beats/min.

Bradycardia often occurs as a normal physiological variant, but may be secondary to drug therapy or an underlying disease process. Bradycardia most often presents as an incidental finding in the asymptomatic patient. Bradycardia can also present as fatigue, breathlessness on exertion, pre-syncope, or syncope. Bradycardia may be intermittent or persistent. The site of conduction disturbance may be the sinoatrial node (SA), atrioventricular (AV) node or His-Purkinje system. Immediate management depends upon the degree of hemodynamic compromise, coexisting medical conditions, the site of conduction disturbance, and prognostic implications.

Sinus Bradycardia

Symptoms
- Asymptomatic, incidental finding, especially if nocturnal
- Fatigue
- Exertional dyspnea
- Less commonly, pre-syncope or syncope.

Causes
- Physiological (fit, young patients at rest) in which case it is asymptomatic and a result of heightened vagal tone
- Drug treatment (e.g. beta-blockers)
- Systemic illness (e.g. hypothyroidism, hypothermia)
- Sinus node disease.

Immediate Management
- Assess hemodynamic status (blood pressure, level of consciousness, urine output, signs of heart failure)
- Identify causative factors (drug history, thyroid status, electrolytes, Lyme carditis)
- If hemodynamically compromised: give atropine 1 mg IV
- Temporary pacemaker wire insertion.

Prognosis and Subsequent Management
- Good prognosis
- Irreversible, symptomatic bradycardia may require permanent pacemaker insertion.

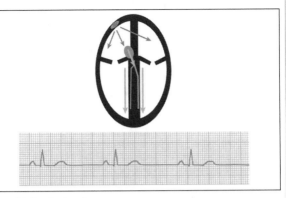

Figure 8.1 Sinus bradycardia.
The P wave and QRS have a constant relationship but the rate is slower than 60 bpm (R–R interval of more than 5 large squares).

Specific Considerations

- Bradycardia arising from sinus or AV nodal disease is typically a stable condition while bradycardia arising from distal conduction system is typically an unstable condition requiring urgent pacing
- Avoid using subclavian access for temporary pacing wire placement to preserve the site in the event a permanent pacemaker will need to be inserted
- Beta-blocker, calcium channel blocker, and digoxin, especially when taken in combination, are common culprits (p. 220–223).

77

Sinus Arrest

Presentation

- Sinus arrest is often intermittent with an adequate rhythm and hemodynamic status in between episodes
- Asymptomatic, coincidental finding, especially if nocturnal (*sinus arrest is only significant if pauses are >3 seconds*)
- Pre-syncope or syncope.

Causes

- Intrinsic sinus node disease
- Carotid sinus hypersensitivity or vasovagal reaction (p. 17).

Immediate Management

- Dictated by presentation frequency and severity of the pauses

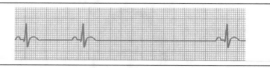

Figure 8.2 Sinus arrest.
The P waves slow or stop suddenly, resulting in a pause. Significant pauses are those >3 seconds, particularly when the patient is awake.

- Stop potentially exacerbating medications (beta-blockers, calcium channel blockers)
- Usually no immediate management is required even though a permanent pacemaker may be indicated
- Very frequent pauses resulting in severe symptoms may require temporary transvenous pacing.

Prognosis and Subsequent Management

- Good prognosis
- Symptomatic sinus arrest may require permanent pacemaker insertion.

Junctional Bradycardia

Junctional bradycardia occurs when the sinus node fails and the AV junction pacemaker takes over. Retrograde P waves (negative in lead II) may be visible immediately before, within, or after the QRS complex, which is usually narrow but may be broad when an IVCD is present (EKG p. 260). Symptoms result from a bradycardia and/or loss of sequential atrial contribution to ventricular filling.

Presentation

- Asymptomatic, incidental finding, especially if nocturnal
- Fatigue
- Exertional dyspnea
- Less commonly, pre-syncope or syncope.

Causes

- Drug treatment (e.g. beta-blockers, calcium channel blockers)
- Systemic illness (e.g. hypothyroidism, hypothermia)
- Hypokalemia
- Sinus node disease with junctional escape.

Immediate Management

- Assess hemodynamic status (blood pressure, level of consciousness, urine output, signs of heart failure)

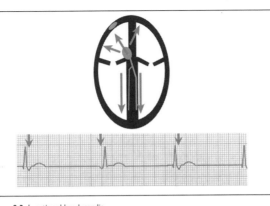

Figure 8.3 Junctional bradycardia.
If the sinus node pacemaker fails, the AV junction is next in line in the pacemaker hierarchy. P waves originate from the AV node area and are therefore negative in leads II, III, and aVF. They occur just before, during, or after the QRS (arrows), depending upon which point in the AV junction they originate. There is a QRS complex, usually narrow, for every P wave.

- Identify causative factors (drug history, thyroid status, electrolytes)
- If hemodynamically compromised: give atropine 1 mg IV.

Prognosis and Subsequent Management

- Good prognosis
- Irreversible, symptomatic bradycardia may require permanent pacemaker insertion.

Specific Considerations

Temporary transvenous pacing for junctional bradycardia may be required for severe hemodynamic compromise. Single chamber ventricular pacing may not improve cardiac output and atrial or dual chamber AV sequential pacing may be required (p. 251).

Atrioventricular Block

Conduction delay or block between the atria and the ventricles may be within the AV node (usually narrow QRS complex, benign, and improves with increase in sympathetic tone or atropine) or the His-Purkinje system (QRS usually wide, worse prognosis and doesn't respond to increase in sympathetic tone or atropine).

Classification

1° AV block

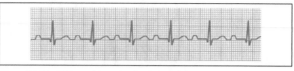

Figure 8.4 The PR interval is greater than 200 ms (1 large square). There is a QRS after every P wave.

2° AV block (EKG p. 261)
Mobitz Type I

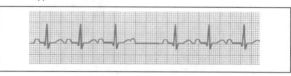

Figure 8.5 The PR interval lengthens after each successive P wave until finally one P wave is not conducted. (Also known as a Wenckebach block.)

Mobitz Type II

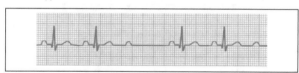

Figure 8.6 P waves fail to conduct to the ventricle in a fixed ratio without preceding lengthening or variation in the PR interval.

3° (complete) AV block (EKG p. 261)

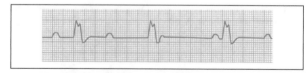

Figure 8.7 All P waves fail to conduct to the ventricle, resulting in a slow, dissociated ventricular escape rhythm. QRS complexes may be narrow or wide depending upon the site of the escape rhythm origin.

Presentation

- Asymptomatic, coincidental finding
- Fatigue, exertional dyspnea, or low cardiac output state
- Pre-syncope or syncope.

Causes

- High vagal tone (this is usually benign and asymptomatic, and usually has a narrow complex escape rhythm.)
- Primary conduction tissue disease
- Myocardial disease (ischemia, infarction, fibrosis, infiltration). This usually affects His-Purkinje system and had a wide complex escape rhythm
- Congenital
- Drugs (e.g. beta-blocker and calcium channel blocker combination).

Immediate Management

1 degree and Mobitz type I 2 degree (Wenckebach) block do not normally require urgent intervention. Mobitz type II and complete AV block may require temporary transvenous pacing.

- Treat any precipitating causes (acute MI, drug overdose, abnormal electrolytes)
- Atropine (1 mg IV), intravenous isoprenaline or other sympathomimetic drugs will improve AV node conduction in the setting of high vagal tone but will have little effect on conduction disturbances due to His-Purkinje disease
- Temporary pacing is required for Mobitz type II 2 degree block or complete heart block with a wide complex escape rhythm, especially if there is a low cardiac output state, reduced perfusion or recurrent syncope
- Complete heart block with a narrow complex QRS and which is asymptomatic may be observed until permanent pacing is performed
- Prognosis and subsequent management
- Discontinue exacerbating antiarrhythmic medications
- There is a good prognosis if the block is due to AV nodal block (narrow QRS, escape rhythm >45 bpm) and reversible cause
- Irreversible Mobitz type II 2 degree block or complete heart block due to His–Purkinje disease has an increased mortality and usually requires permanent pacemaker insertion, whether symptomatic or not.

Box 8.1 Myocardial Infarction and AV Block

Inferior MI

In the setting of acute inferior MI, thrombolysis or primary angioplasty should not be delayed by complete heart block unless the patient is severely hemodynamically compromised. Heart block is usually transient and reperfusion often results in restoration of normal conduction. If conduction returns to normal within

Box 8.1 (Continued)

48 hours, permanent pacemaker insertion is not usually required. Temporary pacing is rarely required and occasionally recovery of AV conduction can take over a week.

Anterior MI

Complete heart block in the setting of acute anterior MI carries a poor prognosis and insertion of a temporary transvenous pacing wire should be considered.

Atrioventricular Block and AF or Flutter

High grade AV block may result in symptoms due to a slow ventricular response, either persistent bradycardia or symptomatic pauses. Pauses (R–R intervals) of less than 3 seconds are not significant (particularly at night).

Causes

- Intrinsic conduction tissue disease
- Coexisting cardiac disease (ischemia, infarction, fibrosis, infiltration)
- Drugs (particularly the combination of beta-blockers and calcium channel blockers).

Immediate management

- Treat any precipitating causes (acute MI, drug overdose, abnormal electrolytes)
- Atropine (1 mg IV) will improve AV node conduction in the setting of high vagal tone but will have little effect on conduction disturbances due to His-Purkinje disease
- Temporary pacing is required only if there is a low cardiac output state with reduced perfusion or recurrent syncope. Slow ventricular rates with mild or infrequent symptoms may be observed until permanent pacing is performed.

Prognosis and subsequent management

- Discontinue exacerbating antiarrhythmic medications
- Irreversible high grade AV block due to His-Purkinje disease has an increased mortality and usually requires permanent pacemaker insertion, whether symptomatic or not.

Tachycardia

Tachycardia is a heart rate of more than 100 beats/min. It is usually subdivided into:
- Narrow complex (regular, QRS duration <120 ms)
- Broad complex (regular, QRS complex >120 ms)

- AF with rapid ventricular response (irregular rhythm, may be narrow or broad complex).

Diagnosis should always be made using a 12-lead EKG, not a telemetry strip, since a true wide complex tachycardia may appear narrow in some leads.

Look for hemodynamic compromise—a decreased level of consciousness, hypotension, pulmonary edema, cardiac ischemia, and poor perfusion. If any of these are present, you should immediately restore sinus rhythm with cardioversion under sedation (if needed).

Look for an underlying cause that may need urgent treatment, such as an acute myocardial infarction, acute pulmonary embolism, or severe electrolyte abnormalities.

EKG Diagnosis of Broad Complex Tachycardia

Any broad complex tachycardia should be assumed to be VT until proven otherwise.

The following EKG criteria confirm a diagnosis of VT:

- *AV dissociation:* Manifests as independent P wave activity, fusion beats or capture beats (EKG p. 264). Be aware that slow VT, or idiopathic VT in a young person, may have 1:1 conduction in a retrograde manner into the atrium
- *QRS duration >160 ms:* However, VT originating from the intraventricular septum may be relatively narrow with QRS 130–150 ms
- *Superior axis* (−45° to −135°) and RBBB-type QRS shape
- *Inferior axis* (60° to 120°) and LBBB-type QRS shape
- The time from the onset of the R wave to deepest point of S wave >100 ms in any chest lead
- *Concordance* across the chest leads (all QRS complexes predominantly positive or predominantly negative).

A prior EKG in sinus rhythm is helpful if it demonstrates bundle branch block that is identical to the wide complex tachycardia QRS shape.

Clinically, the rate and the degree of hemodynamic compromise are not good discriminators.

The presence of structural heart disease and/or a history of ischemic heart disease are strong predictors of a diagnosis of VT.

If in doubt, it is safer to mistreat an SVT as VT rather than treat a VT as an SVT.

The Role of Intravenous Adenosine

Adenosine is a very short-acting intravenous drug that specifically blocks the specialized conducting tissue of the AV node, with lesser effects on the sinus node and atrial myocardium. Its principal effect is to cause transient AV nodal block. Any tachycardia dependent on AV node conduction will therefore terminate when AV node block

83

occurs. Tachycardias that are not dependent on AV node conduction for their maintenance (such as AF, flutter) will continue, although the EKG appearance may transiently change, aiding diagnosis. Some ectopic atrial tachycardias and idiopathic VTs may however also be terminated with adenosine. Likewise, on rare occasions, AV nodal dependent arrhythmias may terminate, but reinitiate after a few beats of sinus rhythm. Adenosine administration often results in ventricular ectopy but it is rare for it to provoke sustained VT.

Administration

Always record a continuous EKG immediately before, during, and after adenosine administration. Administer the adenosine as a rapid IV bolus through a large cannula placed as centrally as possible. This should be followed immediately by a flush of 10 cc of saline.

It is best to connect the adenosine and flush syringes to the cannula through a three-way tap to facilitate administration. Start with

Table 8.1 Tachycardia	
Arrhythmia	**Effect of Adenosine**
Sinus tachycardia	Transient slowing of sinus rate. Transient AV block with ongoing P waves. As adenosine wears off sinus tachycardia rate may increase.
Atrial tachycardia	60% will show transient AV block with ongoing P waves. In some cases the atrial rate may also transiently slow. 10% of automatic atrial tachycardias are adenosine sensitive and will terminate. No effect in the remainder.
Atrial fibrillation	Transient AV block. Fibrillatory baseline still visible up until AV conduction returns.
Atrial flutter	Transient AV block. Flutter waves become clearly visible up until AV conduction returns.
AV nodal re-entrant tachycardia	Tachycardia terminates and sinus rhythm returns.
AV re-entrant tachycardia	Tachycardia terminates and sinus rhythm returns.
Atrial fibrillation and pre-excitation through accessory pathway	QRS complexes transiently widen and ventricular rate may increase further, possibly resulting in ventricular fibrillation.
Ventricular tachycardia	Usually no effect, however some idiopathic ventricular tachycardias in normal hearts may terminate.

a 6 mg bolus, and if there is no effect, increase to 12 mg. Tell the patient to expect transient chest tightness, sweating, and flushing during administration.

Contraindications

- Severe asthma (adenosine is reported to be safe in mild asthmatics)
- Dipyridamole use (inhibits adenosine uptake and potentiates its effect)
- Adenosine should be used with caution in patients with severe sinus node disease, and those who are cardiac transplant recipients
- To reverse the effects of adenosine, give aminophylline IV. Because of the very short half life of adenosine, this is very rarely needed.

Sinus Tachycardia

Sinus tachycardia is a physiological response, usually to physical or emotional stress. The rate is typically 100–160 bpm and is not constant but has subtle variation. There is almost always an identifiable underlying cause. Inappropriate sinus tachycardia is a rare condition marked by a dramatic increase in heart rate with minimal exertion and a mean resting rate >100 bpm. Sinus node re-entrant tachycardia is also rare and may mimic sinus tachycardia but often has a sudden onset and termination and responds to IV adenosine.

Principal Causes

- Pain
- Anxiety
- Sepsis
- Hypoxia (asthma, PE, pulmonary edema)
- Shock
- Anemia
- Inotrope infusions
- Thyrotoxicosis.

EKG Diagnosis

At rapid rates the P wave may be hard to identify, but there are often discrete P waves that are the same shape as those present in sinus rhythm (positive in lead II). There is usually a normal PR interval and 1:1 conduction to the ventricles.

Treatment

Identify and treat the underlying cause.

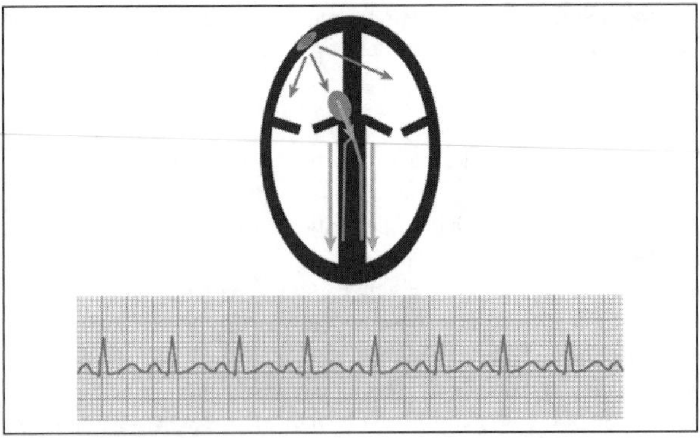

Figure 8.8 Sinus tachycardia.
The P wave is a normal shape and axis and precedes each QRS with a normal PR interval. There are often subtle variations in the heart rate.

Atrial Fibrillation (AF)

This is the most common clinical arrhythmia, affecting 1% of the population. Symptoms result from a rapid, irregular ventricular rate and a loss of the atrial contribution to ventricular filling and cardiac output. Patients may be asymptomatic, have palpitations, chest pain, dyspnea, pre-syncope, syncope, or frank pulmonary edema. AF may be *paroxysmal* (will spontaneously revert to sinus rhythm), *persistent* (requires pharmacologic or electrical cardioversion to restore sinus rhythm) or *permanent* (in which sinus rhythm cannot be restored). The thromboembolic risk that results from the development of AF and the restoration of sinus rhythm must be considered when assessing the various treatment strategies. A left atrial thrombus results from the loss of atrial contractility and increased stasis and pooling of blood in the left atrial appendage. With the restoration of sinus rhythm there is a return to normal atrial contractile function, and this may result in embolism of any atrial thrombus present. This risk should be considered the same whether electrical or pharmacological cardioversion has occurred.

Principal Causes

Age, idiopathic, hypertension, mitral valve disease, cardiomyopathy (ischemic, dilated, or hypertrophic), acute infection, thyrotoxicosis, post-surgery.

EKG Diagnosis

Irregular ventricular rhythm. No discrete atrial activity (although lead V1 often has a coarse, rapid fibrillatory baseline). EKG p. 261.

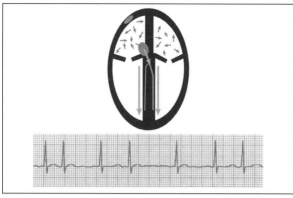

Figure 8.9 AF.
Irregular QRS complexes. No obvious discrete P wave activity.

Treatment—General Principles

The two principal strategies are the restoration of sinus rhythm or ventricular rate control. Some pharmacological treatments may address both. If the duration of AF is greater than 48 hours there is an increased thromboembolic risk associated with restoration of sinus rhythm. In these cases, or in higher stroke risk patients, cardioversion should only be performed if the patient is on long-term effective anticoagulation, or has had a transesophageal echocardiogram to exclude left atrial thrombus, or is hemodynamically compromised such that the benefits of cardioversion outweigh the thromboembolic risks.

If patients present with shorter than 48 hours of AF, the dilemma is between waiting to see if AF stops spontaneously, or using an antiarrhythmic medication or immediate cardioversion before the 48-hour time limit is reached. As long as systemic anticoagulation is started with heparin, there is time to assess the patient and make a decision based upon symptoms, hemodynamic status, and general practicalities. If the duration of AF is unknown, assume it is greater than 48 hours.

AF with Severe Hemodynamic Compromise

Look for a ventricular rate >150 bpm, hypotension and hypoperfusion, reduced conscious level, pulmonary edema, cardiac ischemia. Treatment is with

- Oxygen
- Heparin IV (start at 80 units/kg followed by 18 units/kg/h)
- Immediate synchronized DC shock, or (under sedation if the patient's condition permits more time) using 200–360 J monophasic or 150–200 J biphasic energy.

Symptomatic AF with Mild-Moderate Hemodynamic Compromise

Ventricular rate 100–150 bpm, breathless and/or mild hypotension. Consider other causes for hemodynamic compromise, e.g. sepsis.

Onset <48 hours

- Heparin (start at 80 units/kg followed by 18 units/kg/h), or low molecular weight heparin.
- Consider pharmacological cardioversion with amiodarone (150 mg IV bolus followed by 1 mg/kg/h drip over 6 hours followed by a 0.5 mg/min maintenance drip).
- If the patient has good hemodynamics, no pulmonary edema, and no known structural heart disease (no previous ischemic heart disease or valve disease and a normal transthoracic echocardiogram) an alternative to amiodarone is flecainide 150–300 mg po. Plan for electrical cardioversion 2–3 hours later if drug treatment fails.
- Synchronized DC shock under sedation using 200–360 J monophasic or 150–200 J biphasic energy.
- If immediate electrical cardioversion is not available, start treatment with amiodarone while waiting.

Onset >48 hours

- Heparin (start at 80 units/kg followed by 18 units/kg/h), or low molecular weight heparin.
- Rate control with one of the following:
  - Digoxin 500 mcg in 0.9% saline IV over 1 hour or 500 mcg orally at 12 hourly intervals for three doses, then 125–250 mcg daily
  - Beta-blocker, e.g. metoprolol 25–50 mg po bid
  - Verapamil 40–80 mg po tid
  - Diltiazem sustained release 60–120 mg po bid
  - Amiodarone is poorly effective at rapidly controlling rate in AF when given orally, but can be given as an IV bolus (150 mg) followed by an IV drip at 1 mg/kg/h over 6 hours followed by 0.5 mg/kg/h maintenance drip (then switch to 400 mg po tid for 7 days).
  - Digoxin and amiodarone are the drugs of choice for patients with known structural heart disease and impaired left ventricular function
- Use caution when combining diltiazem or verapamil with beta-blockers.

Minimally Symptomatic AF with No Hemodynamic Compromise

In this setting there is a ventricular rate of less than 100 bpm, together with good perfusion.

Onset <48 hours
- Low-molecular weight heparin.
- Consider antiarrhythmic medication to minimize the risk of recurrent AF post DC cardioversion. It also may restore normal sinus rhythm without the need for cardioversion.
- DC cardioversion can be considered within 48 hours of onset or electively after adequate anticoagulation.

Onset >48 hours
- Anticoagulation and rate control (if required) initially.
- Antiarrhythmic therapy may be required to facilitate elective cardioversion (once anticoagulated) or to control excessive tachycardia during exertion.

Subsequent Management
- Echocardiography to look for underlying heart disease
- Consider anticoagulation with warfarin, especially if structural heart disease, age >75, hypertension, congestive heart failure, DM, prior stroke or other risk factors for stroke, or if planning outpatient cardioversion in 4 weeks time
- Future antiarrhythmic strategy to prevent recurrence if previous episodes or presentation with compromising AF.

Special Considerations for AF
- Attempt to restore NSR sooner rather than later as AF becomes more difficult to suppress when allowed to persist for an extended period of time
- Antiarrhythmic agents are often necessary to maintain NSR over an extended period of time
- Every antiarrhythmic agent has the potential for toxicity and side effects and therefore should be selected, dosed, and monitored carefully
- Rapid control of ventricular rate in the emergency department or ICU setting may also be achieved with a continuous infusion of the IV beta-blocker esmolol. This has the advantage of being short-acting and can be titrated up and down depending upon heart rate and blood pressure response
- Digoxin as a sole agent can slow the resting ventricular rate, but its effect may be lost once the patient becomes active and mobile
- Radiofrequency ablation of AF is performed by electrically isolating the pulmonary veins from the left atrium. When successful, the procedure can provide long-term relief from the symptoms associated with AF.

Box 8.2 **Pre-excited Atrial Fibrillation**

Pre-excited AF (p. 262) conducted through an accessory pathway (a very rapid, irregular, broad complex tachycardia producing severe symptoms) should be treated immediately with either DC cardioversion or antiarrythmic agents that slow conduction over the accessory pathway (e.g., procainamide). Avoid drugs that block AV node conduction (e.g. digoxin, verapamil, and adenosine). All such patients should be referred for radiofrequency ablation to reduce the risk of sudden cardiac death.

Atrial Flutter

Atrial flutter is a macro-reentrant atrial tachycardia with an electrical wavefront that typically rotates around the tricuspid valve, although other less common circuits may present as atypical flutters. Like AF, atrial flutter may be paroxysmal, persistent, or permanent.

The typical atrial flutter circuit is restricted to the right atrium and the rest of the heart is activated passively. The atrial rate is usually a regular 280–320 beats per minute, with the ventricles activated in a 2:1 fashion due to the filtering effect of the AV node. Higher degrees of AV block may occur spontaneously or with the addition of drug therapy. Rarely, 1:1 conduction may occur, leading to extremely rapid ventricular rates and severe symptoms. Symptoms result from the rapid ventricular rate and loss of atrial contribution to ventricular filling and cardiac output. Patients may be asymptomatic, have palpitations, chest pain or dyspnea, pre-syncope, syncope, or frank pulmonary edema. As with AF, the thromboembolic risk needs to be considered when considering the various treatment strategies.

Principal Causes

- Idiopathic
- Hypertension
- Mitral valve disease
- Cardiomyopathy (ischemic, dilated, or hypertrophic)
- Acute infection
- Post-operative

EKG Diagnosis

Typical atrial flutter has a 'saw tooth' baseline with flutter waves at 300 bpm with mainly negative deflections in leads II, III, and aVF. When there is 2:1 conduction to the ventricle, flutter waves may be hard to see as alternate flutter waves are hidden in the QRS complex. The ventricular rate is usually regular at approximately 150 bpm (see the EKG on p. 262).

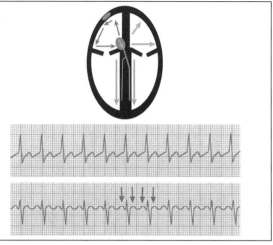

Figure 8.10 Atrial flutter.
Regular QRS complexes, typically at 150 bpm. Rapid, regular atrial activity usually between 280 and 320 bpm (one flutter wave every large square). During 2:1 AV conduction alternate flutter waves may be hidden in QRS complexes. Lead V1 is often a good lead for spotting atrial activity (arrows). In typical flutter the flutter waves are negative in leads II, III and aVF (sawtooth pattern).

Treatment

Two strategies are available (as for AF)—either the restoration of sinus rhythm, or ventricular rate control. Some pharmacological treatments may address both. The treatment strategy should be based on hemodynamic compromise and thromboembolic risk.

Atrial Flutter with Severe Hemodynamic Compromise

Ventricular rate >150 bpm or 1:1 conduction, hypotension and hypoperfusion, pulmonary edema, cardiac ischemia.

- Oxygen
- Heparin (start at 80 units/kg followed by 18 units/kg/h), or low molecular weight heparin
- Synchronized DC shock under sedation (if there is time) using 200–360 J or equivalent biphasic energy.

Symptomatic Atrial Flutter with Mild-Moderate Hemodynamic Compromise

2:1 conduction, breathless and/or mild hypotension.

Onset <48 hours

- Heparin (start at 80 units/kg followed by 18 units/kg/h), or low molecular weight heparin.

- Pharmacological cardioversion with amiodarone 300 mg IV over 1 hour
- Synchronized DC shock under sedation
- 200–360 J or equivalent biphasic energy.

Onset >48 hours

- Subcutaneous low molecular weight heparin
- Rate control with one of the following:
  - Digoxin 500 mcg in 0.9% saline IV over 1 hour or 500 mcg orally at 12 hourly intervals for three doses, then 62.5–250 mcg daily
  - Beta-blocker, e.g. metoprolol 25–50 mg po bid
  - Verapamil 40–80 mg po tid
  - Diltiazem sustained release 60–120 mg po bid
  - Amiodarone is poorly effective at rapidly controlling rate in atrial flutter when given orally but can be given as amiodarone 300 mg IV over 1 hour (then consider 1200 mg over 24 hours given centrally) and then 400 mg tid orally for 7 days. Amiodarone may result in cardioversion so should be avoided in inadequately anticoagulated patients
  - Digoxin and amiodarone are the drugs of choice for patients with known structural heart disease and impaired left ventricular function. Amiodarone may restore sinus rhythm.

Minimally Symptomatic Atrial Flutter with No Hemodynamic Compromise

Ventricular rate <100 bpm, good perfusion.

Onset <48 hours

- Heparin (start at 80 units/kg followed by 18 units/kg/h), or low molecular weight heparin.
- Restore sinus rhythm as for AF with amiodarone or DC cardioversion.
- A strategy to observe and wait for spontaneous cardioversion may also be adopted providing anticoagulation is started.

Onset >48 hours

- Consider anticoagulation.
- Consider the addition of antiarrhythmic to facilitate elective cardioversion once anticoagulated, or to improve rate control during exertion.

Subsequent Management

- Echocardiography to look for underlying heart disease
- Consider anticoagulation with warfarin, especially if structural heart disease, age >70, other risk factors for stroke, cardioversion performed when flutter present for >48 hours, or if planning outpatient cardioversion in 4 weeks time.

- Antiarrhythmic agents do not typically control atrial flutter well; the preferred course is radiofrequency ablation which is highly successful and low risk, to a low risk strategy to prevent recurrence.

Special Considerations for Atrial Flutter

Flecainide should not be given to patients in atrial flutter without additional AV nodal blocking drugs (e.g. beta-blockers).

- Flecainide and other Class 1C drugs may slow the flutter rate within the atrium, allowing 1:1 conduction through the AV node and a paradoxical increase in ventricular rate with worsening of symptoms
- Digoxin has less of an effect in atrial flutter that in AF
- Digoxin, verapamil, and adenosine should be avoided in AF or flutter where there is also ventricular pre-excitation as they may increase conduction through the accessory pathway.

Atrial Tachycardia

- Sometimes called 'ectopic' or 'focal' atrial tachycardia and results from a discrete focus firing automatically at a rate greater than the sinus node. Common sources of tachycardia are the pulmonary veins in the left atrium and the crista terminalis in the right atrium. The ventricle is often activated in a 1:1 fashion unless the atrial rate is particularly fast (>200 bpm) or AV nodal blocking drugs are being used.
- Symptoms result from the rapid ventricular rate and usually manifest as palpitation, dyspnea, pre-syncope, or chest pain.

Principal Causes

In children and young adults the heart is often structurally normal. In older patients it is most likely to be associated with structural heart disease. It may often occur in the setting of an acute illness or trauma (sepsis, surgery, injury).

EKG Diagnosis

There are discrete P waves on the EKG, usually of a different shape to the P waves present in sinus rhythm. There is often a normal PR interval with 1:1 or 2:1 conduction to ventricles. This may be categorized as a 'long RP tachycardia' (i.e., the P to R wave is shorter than the R wave to next P wave) (see the EKG on p. 262).

Treatment

Treatment should be addressed to any underlying cause (infection, trauma, etc).

Severe Hemodynamic Compromise

- Restore sinus rhythm with synchronized DC 200–360 J shock under sedation (if there is time.)
- If the underlying cause is still present, however, there is a high chance of recurrence. Start amiodarone (oral or IV).

Mild Hemodynamic Compromise

In these cases there is a normal Echo and/or no history of structural heart disease

- Beta-blocker, e.g. metoprolol 25–100 mg tid orally
- Verapamil 40–120 mg tid orally
- Amiodarone 300 mg over 1 hour IV then 400 mg tid orally
- Digoxin 500 mcg in 0.9% saline IV over 1 hour or 500 mcg orally at 12 hourly intervals for three doses, then 62.5–250 mcg daily

In cases of sepsis, hypotension or structural heart disease

- Beta-blocker, e.g. metoprolol 25–100 mg tid orally (if structural heart disease but no hypotension or heart failure)
- Amiodarone 300 mg over 1 hour IV then 400 mg tid orally
- Digoxin 500 mcg in 0.9% saline IV over 1 hour or 500 mcg orally at 12 hourly intervals for three doses, then 62.5–250 mcg daily.

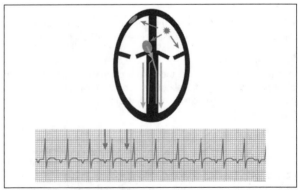

Figure 8.11 Atrial tachycardia.
A focal, automatic tachycardia producing a discrete P wave, although the shape is usually different from the P wave shape seen during sinus rhythm. Usually 1:1 AV conduction unless a very rapid atrial rate or drugs have been given. May have subtle variations in heart rate. Black arrows indicate a compulsory part of the rhythm/circuit; grey arrows indicate bystander (non-participating) pathways.

Atrioventricular Nodal Re-entrant Tachycardia (AVNRT)

AVNRT is the most common form of junctional re-entrant tachycardia in adulthood, and is most often seen in a structurally normal heart. The AV node is a critical component of the re-entrant circuit. It may present at any age and be sustained or non-sustained. The heart rates are typically between 150 and 250 bpm. In the typical form, the atria and ventricles are depolarized (and therefore contract) simultaneously. This atrial contraction against closed AV valves can result in rapid, visible pulsation of the neck veins. The usual symptoms are rapid palpitations with sudden onset and termination, dyspnea, chest tightness, and pre-syncope.

Principal Causes

Attacks may be precipitated by exertion and physical or emotional stress, but are often spontaneous with no obvious cause.

EKG Diagnosis

There is a narrow complex tachycardia, although it may be broad complex if there is bundle branch block or rate-related aberrancy (typical RBBB or LBBB morphology will be present). Simultaneous atrial and ventricular depolarization means the P waves are usually hidden in the QRS and are not visible. In lead V1 the P wave may appear as a 'pseudo-R' wave at the end of the QRS complex (see the EKG on p. 263).

Treatment

- Tachycardia terminates if the AV node can be transiently blocked:
  - Vagal maneuvers: carotid sinus massage, Valsalva maneuvers, ocular pressure, ice application
  - Adenosine IV bolus (see pp. 83–84 for dose and administration)
- If the tachycardia reinitiates immediately after adenosine administration, give verapamil 5–10 mg IV slow injection. However, verapamil should not be given if there is known impaired left ventricular function or significant hypotension as it may cause a further fall in blood pressure.
- If 12 mg of adenosine has no effect after being given appropriately, reconsider the diagnosis before giving verapamil
- DC cardioversion (200–360 J) can be performed if pharmacological treatment fails to terminate the tachycardia.

Subsequent Management

- With incessant tachycardia, start verapamil (initially 5–10 mg IV then 40–120 mg TID orally)

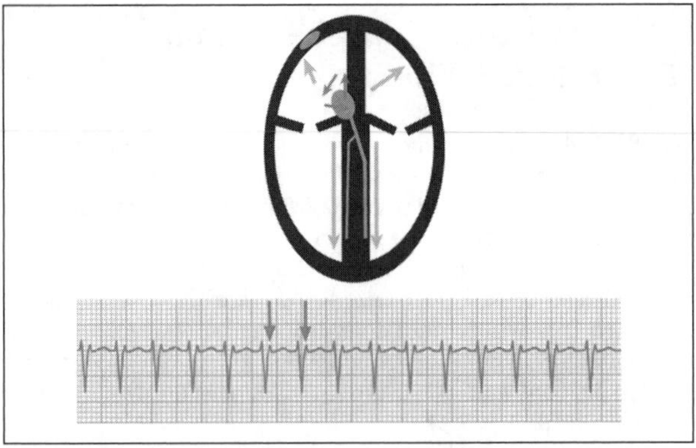

Figure 8.12 AV nodal re-entrant tachycardia.
A rapid, regular tachycardia. Usually narrow complex (unless bundle branch aberrancy occurs). Retrograde P waves occur during the QRS complex and are difficult to see, although typically appear as a 'pseudo-R wave' in lead V1 (arrows). Black arrows indicate a compulsory part of the rhythm/circuit; grey arrows indicate bystander (non-participating) pathways.

- Alternative drug treatments in the emergency setting include esmolol or sotalol IV after consultation with a cardiologist
- First episodes do not usually require prophylactic drug therapy. Maintenance drug therapy or referral for radiofrequency ablation depends upon the frequency, duration, and severity of symptoms.

Atrioventricular Re-entrant Tachycardia (AVRT)

AVRT is the result of an accessory pathway that connects the atria to the ventricles around the tricuspid or mitral valve annuli. The AV node is also a critical component of the re-entrant circuit. Approximately one-third of accessory pathways are able to conduct antegradely from the atrium to the ventricles during sinus rhythm, producing ventricular pre-excitation (Wolff-Parkinson-White syndrome, see the EKG on p. 263). The remaining two-thirds can only conduct retrogradely from ventricles to atria (concealed accessory pathways).

The usual form of tachycardia is conduction from atria to ventricles through the AV node and bundle branches (with normal ventricular depolarization) and conduction from the ventricles to the atria through the accessory pathway (orthodromic reciprocating tachycardia). Antidromic reciprocating tachycardia is much less common and results from antegrade conduction from the atria to the ventricles along the accessory pathway and retrograde conduction up through the AV node. Antidromic tachycardia can therefore only occur in those patients with ventricular pre-excitation.

Patients with Wolff-Parkinson-White syndrome have an increased risk of AF, which if conducted rapidly into the ventricles through the accessory pathway can lead to VF. AVRT is usually seen in structurally normal hearts, although there is an association with Ebstein's anomaly and hypertrophic cardiomyopathy.

Principal Causes and Symptoms

- Attacks may be precipitated by exertion and physical or emotional stress, but are often spontaneous with no obvious cause.
- The usual symptoms are rapid palpitations with a sudden onset and termination, dyspnea, chest tightness, and pre-syncope or rarely syncope.

EKG Diagnosis

There is usually a narrow complex tachycardia, although it may be broad complex if there is bundle branch block or rate-related aberrancy (typical RBBB or LBBB morphology will be present). The retrograde P waves are often visible in the ST segment (see the EKG on p. 263).

Treatment

- As for AVNRT (see p. 95)
- Pre-excited AF (see Box 8.2, p. 90).

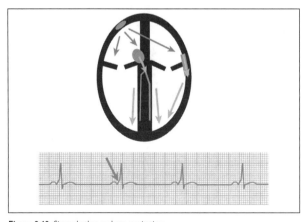

Figure 8.13 Sinus rhythm and pre-excitation.
There is a short PR interval and delta wave at the beginning of the QRS (arrow). Black arrows indicate a compulsory part of the rhythm/circuit; grey arrows indicate bystander (non-participating) pathways.

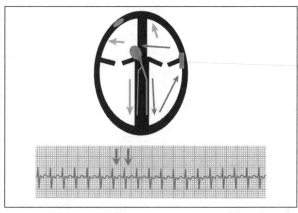

Figure 8.14 Orthodromic tachycardia.
A rapid, regular rhythm. The circuit goes from atrium to ventricle through the AV node and bundle branches so the delta wave disappears and the QRS is narrow (unless there is bundle branch block aberrancy); then from ventricle to atrium through the accessory pathway. The retrograde P wave occurs after the QRS (arrows). Black arrows indicate a compulsory part of the rhythm/circuit; grey arrows indicate bystander (non-participating) pathways.

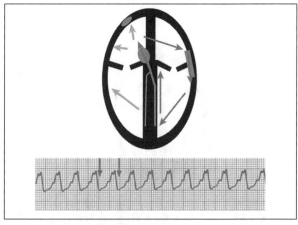

Figure 8.15 Antidromic tachycardia.
Much less common. A rapid, regular rhythm. The circuit goes from atrium to ventricle through the accessory pathway so the ventricle is totally pre-excited and the QRS is very wide; then from ventricle to atrium through the bundle branches and AV node. The retrograde P wave occurs at the end of the QRS (arrows). Black arrows indicate a compulsory part of the rhythm/circuit; grey arrows indicate bystander (non-participating) pathways.

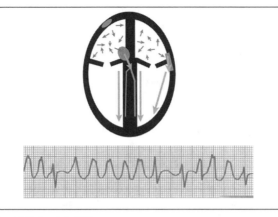

Figure 8.16 Pre-excited AF.
AF is conducted to the ventricles through a combination of the AV node (narrow complexes) and the accessory pathway (wide, pre-excited complexes). The accessory pathway tends to dominate, producing a very rapid ventricular rate. Black arrows indicate a compulsory part of the rhythm/circuit; grey arrows indicate bystander (non-participating) pathways.

Subsequent Management

- As for AVNRT (p. 95)
- In patients with ventricular pre-excitation (Wolff-Parkinson-White syndrome) avoid digoxin and verapamil maintenance therapy, particularly if there is a history of AF. A cardiology consultation is advised for risk stratification.

Ventricular Fibrillation (VF)

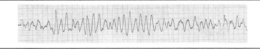

Figure 8.17 Ventricular fibrillation (VF).

- Often a result of ischemic heart disease (acute coronary syndrome, MI)
- Other cardiac precipitants include rapidly conducted AF via an accessory pathway (pre-excited AF p. 90) and ion channel pathologies (Brugada syndrome see p. 265).

- Needs *immediate* defibrillation (p. 268) using standard Advanced Life Support algorithms (p. 269)
- If VF is resistant to attempts at defibrillation then consider giving amiodarone 300 mg IV and using a different defibrillator
- Treat reversible causes—correct K^+, Mg^{2+}
- Repeated episodes of VF (electrical storms) require a consultation with an electrophysiologist (p. 104).

Ventricular Tachycardia (VT)

- VT is usually a re-entrant arrhythmia that results from diseased or scarred myocardium
- Typically, patients have a history of ischemic heart disease or non-ischemic cardiomyopathy, although it may also occur in the setting of acute myocardial ischemia or even the 'normal heart,' where the mechanism may result from automaticity or triggered activity
- The ventricular rate may be anywhere between 100 and 300 bpm with symptoms ranging from none to palpitation, chest pain, and dyspnea, to hemodynamic collapse and cardiac arrest
- Tachycardia may be sustained or non-sustained
- The majority of episodes of VT are monomorphic, i.e., the circuit is consistent and stable and the QRS morphology does not change
- Polymorphic VT results in a beat-to-beat variation in QRS morphology and in the setting of a prolonged corrected QT interval (QT^c) on the sinus rhythm EKG, is called Torsade de Pointes
- Polymorphic VT usually causes collapse and is more often non-sustained although it may sustain and degenerate into VF.

Monomorphic Ventricular Tachycardia

Principal Causes

- Ischemic heart disease (acute or chronic)
- Non-ischemic cardiomyopathies (hypertrophic, dilated, arrhythmogenic right ventricular)
- Idiopathic (fascicular, verapamil-sensitive VT, right ventricular outflow tract VT).

ECG Diagnosis

- Broad complex tachycardia (p. 83 for EKG diagnosis of broad complex tachycardia)

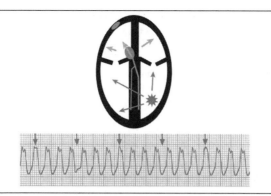

Figure 8.18 Monomorphic ventricular tachycardia.
A regular, wide complex tachycardia. The QRS shape is constant, although may
be distorted by the independent P wave activity if there is visible AV dissociation
(arrows). Black arrows indicate a compulsory part of the rhythm/circuit; grey arrows
indicate bystander (non-participating) pathways.

- Always make the diagnosis on a 12-lead ECG, not a rhythm
  strip
- Idiopathic varieties in normal hearts:
  - Fascicular VT typically has a QRS of 0.12–0.14 ms with RBBB
    and leftward axis morphology
  - Right ventricular outflow tract VT typically has a QRS of
    0.12–0.15 ms with LBBB and inferior axis morphology.

Treatment

- VT that appears to be well tolerated has the potential to
  deteriorate rapidly so all treatments need to be instigated
  promptly, particularly in patients with known or suspected
  impairment of left ventricular function
- Only consider IV adenosine as a diagnostic or therapeutic
  maneuver if the arrhythmia is well tolerated or there is a high
  likelihood of SVT based on history or EKG.

1. VT with Severe Hemodynamic Compromise

- Reduced conscious level, pulmonary edema, cardiac ischemia,
  hypotension with poor perfusion
- Oxygen
- Immediate synchronized DC shock under sedation/general
  anesthesia (200–360 J or equivalent biphasic energy)
- Amiodarone 150 mg IV over 10 minutes through large vein.

2. VT with Mild-Moderate Hemodynamic Compromise

Hypotension with adequate perfusion, mild chest tightness or dyspnea, alert and orientated.

- Oxygen
- Inform anesthetist and prepare for back-up DC cardioversion
- Amiodarone 150 mg IV over 10 minutes through large vein. May be repeated once. Monitor for hypotension
- If BP stable, consider lidocaine 50 mg IV over 2 minutes, repeated every 5 minutes until maximum of 200 mg
- If still VT, synchronized DC shock under sedation/general anesthesia (200–360 J or equivalent biphasic energy).

Subsequent Management of Monomorphic VT

- Identify and treat underlying cause (ischemia, MI)
- Check and replace electrolytes (potassium, magnesium)
- Recurrent episodes of VT require amiodarone or lidocaine infusions and possibly insertion of a temporary transvenous pacing wire for antitachycardia and overdrive pacing (p. 103)
- Consider giving magnesium sulfate (see below)
- Consider ongoing oral drug therapy with amiodarone and/or beta-blockers
- Seek urgent cardiology review (ICD therapy may be indicated).

Polymorphic Ventricular Tachycardia (Torsade de Pointes)

Principal causes are:

- Congenital (long QT syndrome—ask about family history, deafness)
- Drugs (e.g. antiarrhythmics, macrolide antibiotics, tricyclic antidepressants)
- Electrolyte abnormalities (low K^+, low Mg^{2+}).

Hemodynamic collapse is usually present or imminent if the arrhythmia is sustained. Urgent DC cardioversion is indicated.

If conscious and stable, or polymorphic VT is repetitive and non-sustained:

- Check and correct electrolytes (K^+, Mg^{2+})
- If in sinus rhythm the QTc interval is normal, amiodarone 150 mg IV over 10 minutes through large vein. May be repeated once.
- If the sinus rhythm QTc is prolonged (>0.45 seconds) or unknown, give magnesium 1–2 mg in 100 mL 5% dextrose over 2–5 minutes, then 0.5–1 g/hr infusion.

- If necessary, consider lidocaine 50 mg IV over 2 minutes, repeated every 5 minutes until maximum of 200 mg.

Subsequent Management of Polymorphic VT

- Identify and treat underlying cause (electrolytes, ischemia, drugs)
- Potassium should be kept >4.0 mmol/L
- If there is a prolonged QT^c interval in sinus rhythm, especially in the setting of bradycardia, perform pacing with temporary transvenous pacing wire at 90–110 bpm
- Consider isoprenaline infusion (2–10 mcg/min prepared by diluting 1 mg in 500 mL of 5% dextrose) as a temporary measure while awaiting pacing wire insertion
- If normal QT^c interval in sinus rhythm, give oral beta-blockers or amiodarone
- Seek urgent cardiology review.

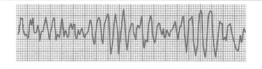

Figure 8.19 Torsade de Pointes.
An irregular, broad complex tachycardia. The QRS axis twists around the baseline.

Box 8.3 **Overdrive Pacing**

- Sustained monomorphic VT may be terminated painlessly by anti-tachycardia pacing in 80–90% of cases
- After positioning a transvenous pacing wire in the right ventricle (p. 251), pacing is performed at a rate 15–20 bpm faster than the VT
- On many temporary pacing boxes there is a '× 3' setting on the rate for this reason
- A high output (5–10 V) may be required
- Capture of the VT is indicated by a change in QRS morphology and an increase in heart rate on the monitor to the pacing rate
- Pacing is abruptly terminated after 5–10 seconds of ventricular capture.

→ There is a risk that acceleration of the VT may occur with degeneration to pulseless VT or VF so operators must be prepared for immediate defibrillation.

Box 8.3 (Continued)

- Once sinus rhythm has been restored, constant background pacing at 90–110 bpm may be performed to prevent recurrent attacks. This is particularly useful with polymorphic VT and a prolonged QT interval, especially in the setting of pauses or bradycardia
- Constant ventricular pacing may result in decreased cardiac output due to the loss of AV synchrony, particularly in the setting of poor left ventricular function. This may be overcome with dual chamber AV sequential pacing.

Electrical Storms

- → Seek early expert cardiology advice.
- VT or VF electrical storms are characterized by multiple, frequent, repetitive episodes of VT or VF
- Episodes may need to be terminated by repeated cardioversion or antitachycardia pacing
- Time, sedation with IV benzodiazepines, IV amiodarone and beta-blockade are the mainstays of treatment
- Correct the correctable (electrolytes, myocardial ischemia, drug intoxication)
- Particular attention should be paid to potassium and magnesium levels
- IV amiodarone should be considered even if the patient has been on oral amiodarone therapy
- Alternative antiarrhythmic therapies include lidocaine or procainamide as an IV infusion (p. 106)
- Beta-blockers (e.g. esmolol, metoprolol) should be initiated as soon as possible
- In addition to pharmacological treatment and insertion of a temporary transvenous pacing wire for overdrive and antitachycardia pacing, patients often require intubation and ventilation to alleviate distress, increase oxygen delivery and reduce the hyperadrenergic state that may accompany repeated cardioversion
- If there is evidence of acute cardiac ischemia, insertion of an intra-aortic balloon pump may increase coronary artery perfusion.

The ICD in the Emergency Department

- Implantable cardioverter defibrillators (ICDs) are programmed to recognize ventricular rates that exceed programmed parameters.

They are able to deliver antitachycardia pacing (which is painless) or shocks (which can be painful) within seconds of the tachycardia commencing

- It is common to program ICDs to attempt antitachycardia pacing for VT that is more likely to be hemodynamically tolerated, e.g. rates between 150 and 180 bpm. Shock therapy will only be delivered if antitachycardia pacing fails or the VT accelerates
- Very rapid VT or VF will often be treated by immediate shock therapy; ICDs are able to deliver up to 6 shocks during a single VT or VF episode, however, if sinus rhythm is transiently restored the counter returns to zero and recommences if VT or VF reinitiates
- During VT or VF electrical storms, ICDs may deliver over 100 shocks within the space of a few hours
- Ventricular rates may also exceed programmed parameters and enter the detection zones in the setting of sinus tachycardia or atrial tachycardias
- Although ICDs try to distinguish between supraventricular tachycardia and VT, if the device is uncertain, it will always assume the worst and treat as if it is VT. Patients may therefore receive inappropriate shocks for sinus or atrial tachycardias with rapid ventricular rates.

One or Two Shocks

Patients who present to the emergency room having received one or two ICD shocks usually do not require hospital admission, particularly if this is not the first time. Providing they are otherwise well, they may be instructed to arrange a visit to their ICD clinic in the next 2–3 days to have device interrogation to check whether the shocks were appropriate.

Multiple Shocks

If the patient has received multiple shocks over a short period of time, they require admission and assessment for electrolyte abnormalities or cardiac ischemia, device interrogation, and often an alteration in antiarrhythmic medication.

Use of a Magnet

ICD shocks may be disabled by placing a magnet over the generator and securing with tape. This may be useful with repetitive inappropriate shocks due to device or lead failure or rapidly conducted atrial arrhythmias. It may also be appropriate as a temporary measure during electrical storms when VT is hemodynamically tolerated but result in frequent painful therapies.

→ The patient must be monitored once a magnet is used as episodes of VF will not be treated by the ICD. The magnet does not disable the bradycardia functions of the ICD.

Commonly Used Antiarrhythmic Agents in the Emergency Setting

Table 8.2 Commonly Used Antiarrhythmic Agents in the Emergency Setting

Drug Name	Dose
Amiodarone	• Cardiac arrest dose 300 mg as IV bolus • Slow IV bolus 150 mg over 10 minutes (in 100–250 mL 5% dextrose) • IV infusion to total 1.2 g in 500 mL 5% dextrose over 24 hours through central line • Oral 200–400 mg tid for 5–7 days then 200 mg maintenance.
Digoxin	• IV loading 0.75–1 mg over 2 hours in 5% dextrose or 0.9% saline • Oral loading 1–1.5 mg 8 hourly over 24 hours • Oral maintenance 62.5–250 mcg daily.
Esmolol	• Urgent IV bolus 1 mg/kg over 30 seconds • IV infusion 10 mg/mL in 5% dextrose or 0.9% saline. Load with 0.5 mg/kg/min for 1 minute only. Maintenance with 0.05–0.3 mg/kg/min, starting at 0.05 mg/kg/min.
Flecainide	• IV 2 mg/kg to a maximum of 150 mg over 15 minutes • Oral 50–150 mg twice daily.
Lidocaine	• IV bolus 50–100 mg over 1–2 minutes • Infusion 4 mg/min for 30 minutes, 2 mg/min for 2 hours, then 1 mg/min.
Magnesium sulfate	• IV bolus 8 mmol (2 mg) over 5–10 minutes in 100 mL 5% dextrose • Infusion 2–4 mmol (0.5–1 g)/h. Concentration should not exceed 20%.

Table 8.2 (Continued)

Drug Name	Dose
Procainamide	• IV 30 mg/min infusion up to a maximum total dose of 17 mg/kg • Maintenance infusion 1–4 mg/min.
Verapamil	• IV 5–10 mg over 2–3 minutes. Additional 5 mg after 5 minutes if necessary • Oral 40–120 mg tid.

Chapter 9

Valve Disease

Acute Valve Problems

Acute valve problems often require urgent treatment, as decompensated heart failure can occur rapidly.

Acute vs. Acute-on-Chronic vs. Cardiac Decompensation

It can sometimes be difficult to differentiate the nature of the current problem, as patients' presentation may be similar:

Acute:	Rapid or sudden deterioration of valve function on previously normal (or near-normal) valves. Nearly always regurgitation. The patient is usually extremely unwell as the LV has not had time to compensate
Acute-on-chronic:	Recent worsening of pre-existing valve dysfunction
Cardiac decompensation:	Pre-existing (and unchanged) valve dysfunction but with left and/or right ventricular decompensation.

Causes

Acute:
- Infective endocarditis
  - leaflet disintegration, perforation or dehiscence (consider an abscess)
  - vegetation (causing incompetence or stenosis)
  - dehiscence of prosthetic valve ring
  - papillary muscle rupture
- Myocardial infarction
  - usually mitral regurgitation from papillary muscle dysfunction (causes: papillary muscle infarction, rupture or tethering to the infarcted myocardial wall)
- Aortic dissection
  - if type A, can dissect into aortic root and cause aortic valve dehiscence and regurgitation
- Ruptured chordae tendinae
  - mitral, or rarely, tricuspid regurgitation
- Trauma

Acute-on-chronic:
Consider all of the above, plus

- Recent deterioration of valve function as part of the natural history
- Severe changes in hemodynamics (e.g. rise or fall in blood pressure, changes in fluid balance).

Cardiac decompensation:

- Natural history, secondary to chronic valve dysfunction
- Changes in hemodynamics (blood pressure changes or fluid shifts)
- Arrhythmias (particularly tachyarrhythmias)
- Other diseases affecting the myocardium (ischemic heart disease, hypertensive heart disease, infiltrative diseases, etc.).

Presentation

The usual symptom is *breathlessness*:

- Acute valve disease — onset over minutes/hours
- Acute-on-chronic — onset over days/weeks (generally)
- Cardiac decompensation — onset over hours–months.

Other symptoms may be:

- Angina (aortic stenosis, acute coronary ischemia)
- Syncope (in aortic or pulmonary stenosis)
- Explosive, tearing back pain in aortic dissection.

Differential diagnosis

→ It is important to look for other causes of breathlessness (p. 10), as even if valve disease is present it may be an innocent bystander. Previous notes/echocardiograms may be helpful in identifying any recent changes. If no change in valve or LV function has occurred, consider other diagnoses.

Clinical signs

- Signs of significant valve disease (see relevant sections below)
- Signs of cardiac failure
- External stigmata of infective endocarditis
- Absent pulses in aortic dissection.

Investigations

Echocardiography

Any patient with a suspected valvular problem presenting acutely needs an echocardiogram. If you suspect true acute valve dysfunction, emergency echocardiography is required. For presentations over days or weeks (i.e., acute-on-chronic or cardiac decompensation), the echocardiogram can usually wait 24–72 hours, depending on the clinical status of the patient—those who are extremely unwell may need an urgent echocardiogram. Transesophageal echocardiography (TEE) may be required for difficult to visualize aortic valves/root, aortic dissection, or mitral regurgitation to assess the feasibility of mitral valve repair.

Chest X-ray
To confirm pulmonary edema or look for other causes of SOB.

EKG
Look for the following:
- Evidence of chronic valve disease (LVH—aortic stenosis/regurgitation; broad P wave—mitral stenosis; AF—mitral stenosis/regurgitation)
- Fast AF or other arrhythmias (these may cause acute decompensation)
- Long PR interval (consider an aortic root abscess)
- Acute MI (consider ischemia)

Blood tests
- CBC—anemia causing or exacerbating SOB; if there is a high WBC consider infection (endocarditis, chest, other)
- Chemistry—look for prerenal azotemia from reduced cardiac output, and a high or low K^+ increasing risk of arrhythmia
- ESR and CRP—infection
- Blood cultures—endocarditis: 3 or 6 sets over 24–48 hours.

General Management
- Identify and treat the cause
- Treat heart failure if present—usually with diuretics (e.g. furosemide 80 mg IV or more) ± vasodilators for regurgitant lesions (ACE inhibitors, or if severe, IV nitrates/sodium nitroprusside, see pp. 63–66)
- Avoid beta-blockers in aortic regurgitation—these lengthen diastole, and may worsen the AR, and also prevent a compensatory tachycardia.

Acute valve regurgitation may require urgent transfer to a tertiary center with cardiothoracic surgical facilities. This should be discussed with the attending cardiologist. These patients are usually very unwell and ICU care is required. They often need emergency valve replacement surgery.

For acute-on-chronic lesions and decompensation, most patients need inpatient referral to a cardiologist for consideration of valve replacement surgery. This may be the first presentation with symptoms, which are important for deciding on surgery. Other lesion-specific advice is given in the relevant sections of this chapter.

Emergency Non-cardiac Surgery (see also p. 214)

If a patient needs emergency surgery and has a concomitant valve lesion, this can sometimes present a problem. In practice, regurgitant lesions are rarely a problem—the afterload reduction from anesthetic agents and hypovolemia tends to reduce any valve leak.

Severe aortic, pulmonary, or mitral stenosis may cause difficulties (but moderate disease is rarely a problem). The lack of capacity to increase cardiac output significantly is the major issue. These patients are at higher operative risk and require careful attention to fluid balance and hemodynamics; large shifts are to be avoided. In some cases, valve replacement surgery may be required prior to the non-cardiac surgery, but the relative risks of valve replacement, delaying the non-cardiac surgery, and proceeding with non-cardiac surgery with appropriate care should be assessed. Non-cardiac surgery for a life-threatening condition should clearly proceed, and the increased risk accepted. This should be discussed with the patient and family (as appropriate) and the content of the discussion should be documented in the medical record.

Remember antibiotic prophylaxis (pp. 117–118).

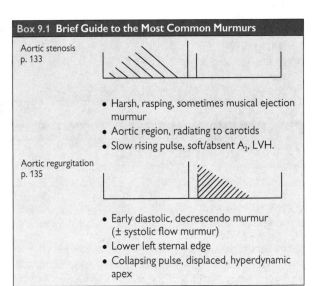

Box 9.1 Brief Guide to the Most Common Murmurs

Aortic stenosis
p. 133

- Harsh, rasping, sometimes musical ejection murmur
- Aortic region, radiating to carotids
- Slow rising pulse, soft/absent A_2, LVH.

Aortic regurgitation
p. 135

- Early diastolic, decrescendo murmur (± systolic flow murmur)
- Lower left sternal edge
- Collapsing pulse, displaced, hyperdynamic apex

Box 9.1 (Continued)

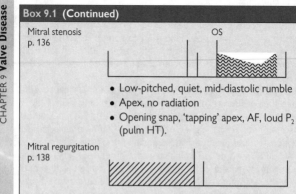

Mitral stenosis
p. 136

OS

- Low-pitched, quiet, mid-diastolic rumble
- Apex, no radiation
- Opening snap, 'tapping' apex, AF, loud P_2 (pulm HT).

Mitral regurgitation
p. 138

- Soft, blowing, monotonous, pansystolic murmur
- Apex, radiating to axilla
- Displaced, hyperdynamic apex.

114

Box 9.2 Grading of Systolic Murmurs

Grade

1 Barely audible
2 Soft but readily detected
3 Prominent
4 Loud, usually with thrill
5 Very loud with thrill
6 So loud, can be heard with the stethoscope just off the chest.

Box 9.3 How to Recognize an Innocent ('Flow') Murmur

- Soft ejection systolic murmur
- Grade ≤2
- Usually heard along left sternal edge/pulmonary region; occasionally at the apex
- Normal heart sounds
- No associated thrills or added sounds
- No signs of LV dilatation
- Normal ECG and no cardiac abnormalities on CXR.
→ Innocent murmurs do not need echocardiography.
→ Diastolic, pan-systolic and loud murmurs (grade 4+) are not 'innocent.'

Indications for Valve Surgery

Emergent (Within Few Hours)

- Acute valve regurgitation with severe heart failure (NYHA 3 or 4)
- Type A aortic dissection ± aortic regurgitation
- Post-infarct mitral regurgitation
- Ruptured sinus of Valsalva aneurysm.

Urgent (Inpatient)

- Rapidly increasing SOB or pulmonary edema with chronic valve lesion
- Unstable prosthetic valve
- Uncontrolled infective endocarditis despite adequate antibiotics:
  - Heart failure due to valve dysfunction
  - Valve obstruction from vegetation/thrombus
  - Fungal and other anti-microbial resistant endocarditis (e.g. *Brucella*, *Coxiella*)
  - Cardiac abscess formation (usually aortic root)
  - Persistent bacteremia (after 7–10 days). This is a relative indication for urgent surgery to be considered.
  - Recurrent emboli. This is a relative indication for urgent surgery to be considered.
  - Large (>10 mm) mobile vegetations (these increase the risk of embolization). This is a relative indication for urgent surgery to be considered.
- Early prosthetic valve endocarditis (<2 months from implantation).

Elective

- Severe aortic stenosis (mean gradient >40 mmHg and AVA of <1.0) *with stable symptoms* of dyspnea, angina, or syncope *or* LV dysfunction (EF <50%)
- Severe mitral stenosis (mean gradient >10 and AVA <1.0) with either class 3 or 4 symptoms or asymptomatic with PAP of >60 or AF and a non-pliable valve not amenable to valvuloplasty
- Severe mitral regurgitation:
  - If any symptoms
  - If asymptomatic with reduced LV function (EF <60%) *or* end-systolic diameter >40 mm
- Severe aortic regurgitation:
  - If symptomatic
  - If asymptomatic with reduced LV function (EF <55%) *or* an end-systolic diameter >50 mm
- Moderate to severe valve disease if other cardiac surgery planned.

Chronic Valve Disease

Most valve lesions are managed conservatively, particularly if patients are well. In the absence of symptoms or progressive LV dysfunction, there is rarely a need for surgery and these patients can be managed in outpatients with follow-up, often on an annual basis. Progression to LV dysfunction or excess dilatation or development of symptoms should prompt consideration of surgery. Mild disease may not need follow up, but does need prophylaxis against endocarditis (see below).

Antibiotic Prophylaxis

Most patients with chronic valve lesions are at risk of endocarditis, and prophylactic antibiotic therapy should be given before dental and surgical procedures where there is significant risk (p. 118).

Infective Endocarditis

This condition still carries a high mortality (15–20%) despite modern antibiotics. Uncomplicated *strep viridans* infections have a better prognosis, but staphylococcal and prosthetic valve endocarditis carry a high mortality. Potential reasons for the continued high mortality are: an aging population, an increased incidence of prosthetic endocarditis, longer lifespan of patients with congenital heart disease, tricuspid valve endocarditis from intravenous drug use, and antibiotic resistance.

Infective endocarditis is most likely to develop where underlying structural cardiac defects are present, which underlines the importance of prevention in susceptible individuals. Endocarditis occurring on normal valves tends to involve the more virulent organisms, especially *Staph. aureus*. Other factors which increase risk are: increased susceptibility to infection (old age, chronic alcoholism, hemodialysis, diabetes, and immunosuppression) and recurrent bacteremia (from inflammatory bowel disease, colon carcinoma, IV drug use).

Prophylaxis

Prophylaxis guidelines have significantly changed with the publication of the AHA/ACC statement in 2006. Only an extremely small number of cases of IE might be prevented by antibiotic prophylaxis even if prophylaxis is 100% effective. Routine dental prophylaxis is no longer warranted as bacteremia resulting from daily activities is much more likely to cause IE than bacteremia associated with a dental procedure. Antibiotic prophylaxis is not recommended based solely on an increased lifetime risk of acquisition of IE. Recommendations for IE prophylaxis have therefore changed in recent years and are now limited to those conditions listed in Box 9.4.

Antibiotic prophylaxis is reasonable for all dental procedures that involve manipulation of gingival tissues or periapical region of teeth or perforation of oral mucosa only for patients with underlying cardiac conditions associated with the highest risk of adverse outcome from IE listed in Box 9.4.

> ### Box 9.4 Patients Who Require Antibiotic Prophylaxis
>
> - Prosthetic cardiac valve or prosthetic material used for cardiac valve repair
> - Previous IE
> - Congenital heart disease (CHD)
>   - Unrepaired cyanotic CHD, including palliative shunts and conduits
>   - Completely repaired congenital heart defect with prosthetic material or device, whether placed by surgery or by catheter intervention, during the first 6 months after the procedure
>   - Repaired CHD with residual defects at the site or adjacent to the site of a prosthetic patch or prosthetic device (which inhibit endothelialization)
> - Antibiotic prophylaxis is no longer recommended for any other form of congenital heart disease
> - Cardiac transplantation recipients who develop cardiac valvulopathy

Antibiotic prophylaxis is only reasonable for procedures on respiratory tract or infected skin, skin structures, or musculoskeletal tissue for patients with underlying cardiac conditions associated with the highest risk of adverse outcome from IE. Antibiotic prophylaxis solely to prevent IE is not recommended for GU or GI tract procedures. Other simple measures are equally important in the prevention of bacteremia, and patients at risk should pay attention to these such as good oral and feet hygiene and attention to cuts and skin disorders which may allow bacteria to penetrate the skin (especially in diabetics).

Antibiotic Regimens

An antibiotic for prophylaxis should be administered in a single dose before the procedure. If the dosage of antibiotic is *inadvertently* not administered before the procedure, the dosage may be administered up to 2 hours after the procedure. Amoxicillin or ampicillin is the preferred agent for methicillin-resistant strain of staphylococcus.

Patients already receiving antibiotics

If a patient is already receiving long-term antibiotic therapy with an antibiotic that is also recommended for IE prophylaxis for a dental procedure, one should select an antibiotic from a different class rather than increase the dosage of the current antibiotic. If possible, it would be preferable to delay a dental procedure until at least 10 days after completion of the antibiotic therapy. This may allow time for the usual oral flora to be reestablished.

Patients receiving parenteral antibiotic therapy for IE may require dental procedures during antimicrobial therapy, particularly if subsequent cardiac valve replacement surgery is anticipated. In these cases, the parenteral antibiotic therapy for IE should be continued and the timing of the dosage adjusted to be administered 30–60 minutes before the dental procedure. This parenteral antimicrobial therapy is administered in such high doses that the high concentration would overcome any possible low-level resistance developed among mouth flora (unlike the concentration that would occur after oral administration).

Patients who undergo cardiac surgery

A careful preoperative dental evaluation is recommended so that required dental treatment may be completed whenever possible before cardiac valve surgery or replacement or repair of CHD. Such measures may decrease the incidence of late prosthetic valve endocarditis caused by *strep viridans*.

Patients who undergo surgery for placement of prosthetic heart valves or prosthetic intravascular or intracardiac materials are at risk for the development of infection. Because the morbidity and mortality of infection in these patients are high, perioperative prophylactic antibiotics are recommended. Prophylaxis at the time of cardiac surgery should be directed primarily against staphylococci and should be of short duration. A first-generation cephalosporin is most often used, but the choice of an antibiotic should be influenced by the antibiotic susceptibility patterns at each hospital. For example, a high prevalence of infection by methicillin-resistant *Staph. aureus* should prompt the consideration of the use of vancomycin for perioperative prophylaxis. The majority of nosocomial coagulase-negative staphylococci are methicillin-resistant. Nonetheless, surgical prophylaxis with a first-generation cephalosporin may be recommended for these.

Prophylaxis should be initiated immediately before the operative procedure, repeated during prolonged procedures to maintain serum concentrations intraoperatively, and continued for no more than 48 hours postoperatively to minimize emergence of resistant microorganisms.

There are insufficient data to support specific recommendations for patients who have undergone heart transplantation. Such patients are at risk of acquired valvular dysfunction, especially during episodes of rejection. Endocarditis that occurs in a heart transplant patient is associated with a high risk of adverse outcome (see table above). Accordingly, the use of IE prophylaxis for dental procedures in cardiac transplant recipients who develop cardiac valvulopathy is reasonable, but the usefulness is not well established. The use of prophylactic antibiotics to prevent infection of joint prostheses during potentially bacteremia-inducing procedures should be discussed jointly with the orthopedic team performing the surgery.

Presentation of Infective Endocarditis

This may be acute, sub-acute, or occasionally hyper-acute:

Sub-acute —insidious onset, usually over months

Acute —presentation over 1–4 weeks

Hyper-acute —rapid deterioration over hours or days, usually due to acute valve regurgitation.

While the classical sub-acute presentation, with months of non-specific malaise, still occurs, there is an increasing tendency towards acute presentations, which may reflect increasing numbers of more virulent organisms, e.g. *Staph. aureus* or the HACEK group (see p. 101).

The presentation is usually with non-specific symptoms and can mimic many other systemic diseases. A high index of suspicion is therefore necessary (see box, opposite). Cardiac tumors can sometimes mimic endocarditis (atrial myxoma) and these should also be considered—but they are very rare.

Clinical Features

These can be divided into four areas, attributable to:

Infection

- Fever
- Night sweats
- General malaise
- Weight loss
- If longstanding: anemia, clubbing, splenomegaly.

Cardiac involvement

- New or altered murmur
- Signs of severe valve regurgitation
- Left ventricular failure due to valve deterioration or direct involvement of the myocardial endothelium
- Prolonged PR interval if aortic root abscess.

Immunological phenomena

- Microscopic hematuria, glomerulonephritis, generalized vasculitis, arthralgia
- Petechiae, splinter hemorrhages in the nail beds, Osler's nodes (tender nodules [infarcts] on finger pulps/palms/soles), Janeway lesions (painless palm/sole erythematous macules)

- Flame/boat-shaped retinal hemorrhages, Roth spots (boat-shaped retinal hemorrhages with pale center).

→ Immunological phenomena tend not to occur in acute presentations, as the infection has evolved too quickly for their development. They also do not occur with right-sided lesions.

Emboli

- Commonly: cerebral, retinal, coronary, splenic, mesenteric, renal
- Pulmonary in right-sided endocarditis
- May develop into abscesses, or a mycotic aneurysm.

Potential routes of infection should also be sought (e.g. teeth, skin infections).

Box 9.5 Murmurs and Endocarditis

- A genuine new murmur in the context of someone who is unwell is highly significant and the old adage 'fever + new murmur = endocarditis until proven otherwise' is true to an extent. In practice however, knowing whether the murmur is new, or a newly discovered old murmur, can be difficult. However, endocarditis does of course occur commonly on valves with pre-existing lesions (i.e. murmurs) and a change in the character of a pre-existing murmur is suspicious. It should also be remembered that any infection will tend to increase cardiac output and can thus lead to an innocent 'flow' murmur, or a slight change in a pre-existing murmur. Overall, the picture is complicated.
- Therefore, murmurs that are more than 'innocent' (see p. 114) in the context of non-specific illness require investigation, though by themselves they are not diagnostic of endocarditis (see also indications for echocardiography below). In particular, the combination of fever plus murmur (either new or old) is not enough for a diagnosis without other supporting evidence, and antibiotics should NOT be started until other evidence is available, unless the patient is very unwell and a presumptive diagnosis of endocarditis is likely. In all cases, 3 or 6 sets of blood cultures should be taken prior to commencing antibiotic treatment.

Box 9.6 Indications for Echocardiography in Suspected Endocarditis

—when level of suspicion is high:
- New valve lesion (usually regurgitant murmur)
- Embolic events of unknown origin
- Sepsis (i.e. bacteremia plus systemic features) of unknown origin

Box 9.6 (Continued)

- Hematuria, glomerulonephritis and suspected renal infarction
- Fever plus:
  - Positive blood cultures for organisms typical for endocarditis
  - High predisposition for endocarditis, e.g. prosthetic valve
  - First manifestation of heart failure
  - Newly-developed conduction disturbance or ventricular arrhythmias
  - Typical immunological manifestations of endocarditis
  - Multifocal/rapidly changing pulmonary infiltrates
  - Peripheral abscesses of unknown origin (e.g. renal, splenic, spinal)
  - Predisposition plus recent diagnostic/therapeutic intervention known to result in significant bacteremia.

NB: *a fever without other evidence for endocarditis is not an indication for echocardiography.*

121

Diagnosis

The cornerstone of diagnosis is microbiological evidence of infection. Although helpful, echocardiography (even TEE) does not exclude endocarditis, and can produce false positive results. It is therefore crucial that an accurate clinical picture is obtained (also to exclude other sources of infection), and that rigorous measures are taken to identify any infective organism—adequate blood cultures are key.

The diagnosis is usually based on a bacteremia with a likely organism, coupled with evidence of cardiac involvement (e.g. a new regurgitant lesion or vegetation). Investigations are therefore aimed at identifying these and also assessing severity and/or complications. There are situations, however, where other features may be helpful in reaching a diagnosis, and the widely accepted Duke criteria for diagnosis (see Table 9.1) include these.

Investigations

Blood cultures

3–6 sets of blood cultures should be obtained: 3 when the patient is very unwell and the diagnosis of endocarditis is likely; 6 when the patient is well and the diagnosis not obvious but suspicion is high. Each set should be taken from a different site and, ideally, spaced at intervals of >1 hour.

Echocardiography

Echocardiography should be performed if there is a high clinical suspicion of endocarditis (see Box 9.6). It is invaluable for diagnosis

and also detection of any complications. Strong identifiers of endocarditis are:

- Characteristic vegetations
- Abscesses
- New prosthetic valve dehiscence
- New regurgitation.

Transthoracic echocardiography (TTE) has high specificity for vegetations (98%) but low sensitivity (60%) and TEE may be required.
Combined TTE and TEE have a high negative predictive value (95%)
but note this is not 100%, and this underlines the importance of good
clinical and microbiological evidence.

- *Native valves:* TTE should be the initial investigation. TEE is
  required when the TTE images are of poor quality, when high
  clinical suspicion remains despite a normal TTE or when a
  prosthetic valve is involved.
- *Prosthetic valves:* TEE is nearly always required for better
  visualization but important information can still be obtained from
  TTE, so it is normal to perform this at the same time, just prior to
  the TEE.

Other investigations

- *Bloods:* CBC—anemia, neutrophilia, ESR, CRP—non-specific but
  raised in 90% of cases of endocarditis, Chemistry—renal function
  (needs regular repeat assessment), serum for immunology for
  atypical organisms.
- *Urinalysis:* Microscopic hematuria ± proteinuria; red cell casts &
  heavy proteinuria if glomerulonephritis.
- *EKG:* Lengthening PR interval (think of an aortic root abscess).

Treatment

General considerations

Treat heart failure and shock as appropriate

- Ensure blood cultures are taken prior to starting antibiotic
  therapy
- Give anti-microbial therapy in adequate doses IV for
  4–6 weeks
- Monitor response to therapy—both clinically and biochemically
- Consider surgery if significant complications arise (see p. 115).

Antimicrobial therapy

- *Uncomplicated cases:* Treatment may be postponed for 48 hours,
  allowing time for initial blood culture results. If the patient has
  had antibiotics within the last week, it is better to wait at least
  48 hours before taking blood cultures.

Table 9.1 Modified Duke Criteria for Diagnosis of Endocarditis

Confirmed diagnosis is based on either:

Pathological criteria:	Organisms or histological evidence of active endocarditis in a vegetation (embolized or not) or intra-cardiac abscess.
Clinical criteria:	2 major criteria, or 1 major and 3 minor criteria, or 5 minor criteria.

Major criteria

Microbiological involvement—either:
- Typical microorganism for endocarditis from two separate blood cultures (Viridans streptococci; *Strep. bovis*; HACEK group*; community acquired *S. aureus/enterococci* in the absence of a primary focus)
- Persistently positive blood cultures with consistent organisms (drawn >12 hours apart, or ≥3 +ve cultures with first and last drawn >1 hour apart)
- Positive serology or molecular biology for Q-fever, *Coxiella burnettii* or other causes of culture-negative endocarditis.

Evidence of endocardial involvement:
- Oscillating intra-cardiac mass (vegetation)
- Abscess
- New partial dehiscence of prosthetic valve
- New valve regurgitation (either clinical or echocardiographic).

Minor criteria
- Predisposing heart condition or IV drug use
- Fever >38.0°C
- Vascular phenomena (arterial emboli, septic pulmonary infarcts, mycotic aneurysm, intracranial or conjunctival hemorrhage, Janeway lesions, splinter hemorrhages, splenomegaly, newly diagnosed clubbing)
- Immunological phenomena (glomerulonephritis, Osler's nodes, Roth spots, +ve rheumatoid factor, high ESR >1.5× normal, high CRP >100 mg/L)
- Microbiological evidence—+ve blood culture not meeting major criterion¶, or serological evidence of active infection with organism consistent with infective endocarditis
- Echocardiography findings consistent with infective endocarditis but falling short of major criterion.

---

* *Hemophilus, Acintobacillus, Cardiobacterium, Eikenella,* and *Kingella sp.*
¶ Excludes single +ve culture for coagulase –ve Staph. and organisms not associated with infective endocarditis.

Reprinted from Durack DT, Lukes AS, Bright DK. New criteria for diagnosis of infective endocarditis: utilization of specific echocardiographic findings: Duke Endocarditis Service. *Am J Med* 1994; 96:200-209, with permission from Elsevier.

- *Severely unwell patients:* Sepsis, severe valve dysfunction, conduction disturbances, embolic events, should have empirical antibiotic therapy (see Table 9.2) after 3 sets of blood cultures have been taken. Treatment can be adjusted once culture results are known.

- *Choice of therapy:* This is guided by the organism but in all cases, microbiological advice should be sought early. Suggested regimens are in the table opposite, but these are for guidance only.
- *Treatment duration:* In general this needs to be prolonged (4–6 weeks) IV therapy in adequate doses. Occasionally, shorter courses may be appropriate for the most sensitive streptococci only (see table). A tunneled central line or peripherally inserted central catheter (PICC line) is usually inserted to facilitate IV therapy and reduce infections and other complications from repeated peripheral cannulae.

Prosthetic valve endocarditis

- Prosthetic (metal) valve endocarditis often requires replacement of the valve. Even then, recurrence rates are high (9–20%). This is due to the difficulty of eradicating infection from prosthetic material. Biological valves may be treated with antibiotics alone but need for surgery is still higher than for native valves
- Even with good a TTE, a TEE is required to visualize the valve properly due to the shadowing effect of the metal
- Prolonged antibiotic therapy is required (6 weeks)
- Warfarin is often replaced with heparin for better control of anticoagulation and potential surgical situations.

Valve replacement surgery in endocarditis (see p. 115)

- 30% require this during the acute episode. Consider surgery if valve function deteriorates enough to cause heart failure, infection remains uncontrolled despite adequate therapy, or significant complications arise
- Although valve replacement surgery during active endocarditis does carry a risk of re-infection of the prosthesis, the risk is low and the risk to the patient (of death or irreversible LV dysfunction) if not operated on is higher for the indications given
- If cerebral emboli/hemorrhage has occurred, surgery should be deferred for 10 days–3 weeks if possible.

Complications (esp. common with *S. aureus*)

Cardiac

- Abscesses (20–40% native valves; 50–100% prosthetic valves)—valve ring, intra-myocardial or pericardial. Usually require valve replacement surgery + debridement of the abscess
- Valve rupture, perforation or regurgitation

Table 9.2 Empirical Treatment for Endocarditis (if essential)

Be guided by the clinical setting:

- Onset over weeks: Benzylpenicillin + gentamicin
- Rapid onset (days) or   Flucloxacillin + gentamicin
  history of skin trauma (likely
  staphylococcus):
- Recent metal valve replacement: Vancomycin + gentamicin + rifampicin

Antibiotic therapy for known organism
—*seek microbiological advice in all cases*
Viridans streptococci and *Strep. Bovis*
- Benzylpenicillin 4–6 weeks + gentamicin 2 weeks.

Staphylococci
- Methicillin-sensitive: Flucloxacillin 6 weeks + gentamicin 3–5 days
- Methicillin-resistant: Vancomycin 6 weeks + gentamicin 3–5 days
- Prosthetic valves: continue gentamicin for 6 weeks and add rifampicin
  6 weeks.

Enterococci/HACEK group (the latter need amoxicillin)
- Benzylpenicillin/amoxicillin 4–6 weeks + gentamicin 4–6 weeks.

Penicillin-allergic patients
- Vancomycin 4 weeks + gentamicin 2 weeks.

Doses

- Benzylpenicillin—for streptococci, relies on minimum inhibitory
  concentration (MIC) of antibiotics required (i.e. sensitivity to penicillin):
  - MIC <0.1 mg/L: 7.2–12 g IV daily in 4–6 divided doses
  - MIC >0.1 mg/L   12–14 g IV daily in 4–6 divided doses (& enterococci):
- Gentamicin: 3–5mg/kg IV daily in 2–3 divided doses (max 240 mg/d)
  —requires blood level checking; dose is reduced in renal failure
- Flucloxacillin: 8–12 g IV daily in 4 divided doses
- Amoxicillin: 12 g IV daily in 4–6 divided doses
- Vancomycin: 30 mg/kg IV daily in 2 divided doses (infused over 2 hours)
- Rifampicin: 300 mg TDS po.

- Sinus of Valsalva rupture (2° to abscess). Requires emergency
  surgery
- Ventricular septal defect (from myocardial abscess rupture)
- LV failure—due to valve dysfunction or direct myocardial
  involvement
- AV heart block—due to aortic root abscess
- Relapse of endocarditis
- Chronic valve regurgitation—if significant regurgitation occurs,
  but not enough to require urgent valve replacement, valve
  replacement may be required in the future (20–40% of cases).
  The indications are the same as for other causes of regurgitation
  (p. 115).

Table 9.3 Shorter Treatment Regimens

May be possible if all the below apply:
- Infection with fully sensitive streptococcus (MIC <0.1 mg/L) on native valve
- Rapid response to treatment within the first 7 days
- Any vegetations on echocardiography <10 mm
- No cardiovascular complications
- Home situation suitable.

Regimes possible
- Benzylpenicillin alone for 2 weeks (rarely, for exquisitely sensitive organisms)
- Benzylpenicillin alone for 1–2 weeks plus further 2 weeks ambulatory (home) treatment with ceftriaxone
- Benzylpenicillin + gentamicin for 2 weeks ± further 2 weeks ambulatory treatment with ceftriaxone.

Non-cardiac

- **Emboli** (20–40%) may cause stroke, peripheral arterial occlusion, or organ infarcts. May also cause abscesses due to infected nature of embolic material. Abdominal abscesses should be operated on prior to cardiac surgery. Splenic abscesses are particularly prone to rupture and splenectomy may be required.
- **Mycotic aneurysms** (2–15%)—often caused by embolized infected material. Common sites: sinuses of Valsalva, cerebral, mesenteric & renal arteries. Intra-cranial aneurysms have a high mortality (60%), and this is increased still further if rupture occurs (causing a subarachnoid hemorrhage: 80% mortality)
- **Renal failure** (sepsis, dehydration, glomerulonephritis, emboli).

Culture Negative Endocarditis (5% of cases)
Causes:

- Previous antibiotic therapy (the most common cause)
- Unusual organism—HACEK group, Brucella, Chlamydia, Coxiella (Q fever), Legionella, Bartonella, Mycobacteria, Nocardia, fungi (Candida, Aspergillus, Histoplasma).

Management

- Consider other (non-cardiac) causes for fever
- If high clinical suspicion for endocarditis remains:
  - Consult with microbiology regarding prolonged or special cultures; take serum for serology of unusual organisms
  - For unwell patients, treat empirically (p. 125)
  - For well patients, await microbiological diagnosis

- If valve replacement surgery is required, the excised valve should be sent for culture and broad spectrum polymerase chain reaction (PCR) for DNA identification of organisms.

Prosthetic Valves

All patients with either bioprosthetic or metallic valves should be on aspirin 75–100 mg daily, even if they are taking Coumadin.

Types

Bioprosthetic

- Obtained from human cadavers (homograft), or manufactured from bovine or porcine pericardium (xenograft; e.g. Carpentier-Edwards). Pericardial valves may be suspended from 3 metal struts (stented valve) or contained within a covered wire frame (stentless)
- Do not require long term anticoagulation. Usually require 3 months of either warfarin or very rarely aspirin alone post-surgery while surfaces endothelialize unless other risk factors are present
- Generally last 10–15 years. For this reason, they are usually implanted in a) older patients, who also tend to be less active, reducing the physical burden on the valve; b) those in whom anticoagulation is contraindicated; and c) young women who may be considering pregnancy.

Metallic

Metallic valves are durable (can last >20 years) but thrombogenic, so all require lifelong anticoagulation. Target INR of 2–3 for aortic bileaflet or Medtronic Hall. For all others target INR is 2.5–3.5. If any embolic events occur the target INR should be increased. There are three main sub-types:

- Ball and cage (e.g. Starr-Edwards) Older style, unlikely to be implanted now. Durable, and long track record, but higher resistance to flow and high thrombogenicity
- Single tilting disc (e.g. Bjork-Shiley, Medtronic Hall)
- Bileaflet tilting disc (e.g. St. Jude). This is the most commonly used today. Good track record, low resistance to flow, and low thrombogenicity.

Clinical Considerations

- Bioprosthetic valves should not sound different from native valves, but pericardial valves may have a flow murmur
- Metallic valves have a distinctive 'click' as the valve either opens or closes. This should be a crisp sound—a dull or indistinct sound suggests thrombus or vegetation on the valve. Although flow

murmurs may occur, these are soft. Other murmurs (pan-systolic, diastolic) suggest regurgitation
- Annual follow-up is routine for patients with prosthetic valves.

Echocardiography

Systolic flow velocities are in general increased with a normally functioning prosthetic valve. Metal prostheses can have high velocities (>3 m/sec) and the normal range for that valve needs to be taken into account. The smaller the valve, the higher the forward velocity.

- *Biological:* Homografts look like normal valves; pericardial valves have a smaller valve ring in general and hence have slightly increased flow velocities, though the newer stentless type look virtually normal and have normal flow velocities
- *Metallic valves* cause echo 'shadows' which limit the available information. TEE may therefore be required on occasions to assess valve function in detail. For tilting-disc valves, it is normal to see tiny regurgitant 'wash' jets.

Prosthetic Valves

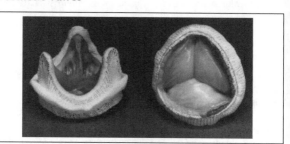

Figure 9.2 Carpentier-Edwards bioprosthetic valve.

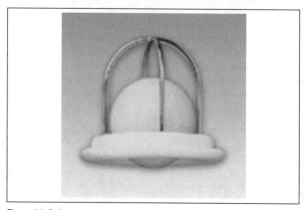

Figure 9.3 Ball and cage valve.

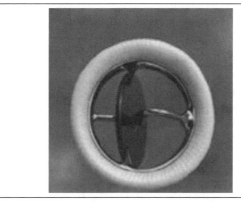

Figure 9.4 Single tilting disc valve.

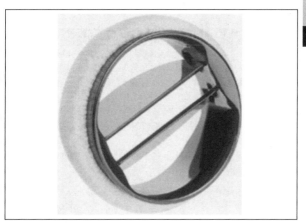

Figure 9.5 Bileaflet tilting valve.

Complications

Thrombosis

This is usually from inadequate anticoagulation. The risk is higher in mitral prostheses. Patients present with heart failure or systemic emboli. Treat with heparin anticoagulation ± thrombolysis, thrombectomy, or valve replacement.

Hemolysis

Small amounts of hemolysis are common with metallic valves. Significant hemolysis is usually secondary to valve dysfunction—paravalvular leak, valve dehiscence, or endocarditis. Blood tests will reveal anemia, an increased reticulocyte count and LDH, and decreased haptoglobins. Urinary hemosiderin present. Treat the anemia with ferrous sulfate (and blood transfusions as required) and also treat the underlying cause; this may require a repeat of the valve replacement surgery, though there are new percutaneous devices for closing paravalvular leaks.

Endocarditis
About 5% patients with prosthetic valves may develop endocarditis. Endocarditis is discussed above (p. 116).

- Early prosthetic valve endocarditis (<2 months post-implantation) is usually due to contamination at the time of surgery or IV cannulae. Common organisms: *S. aureus, S. epidermidis*, gram-negative bacteria, fungi
- Late prosthetic valve endocarditis has similar organisms to native valve endocarditis.

Box 9.7 Anticoagulation for Metal Valves—Acute Issues

In general, the risk of thrombosis on a metal valve without anticoagulation for a few days is low, though should be minimized with heparin where possible.

Emergency surgery
INR can be normalized with fresh frozen plasma to allow emergency surgery. Once stable post-surgery, warfarin can be re-started.

Acute hemorrhage
In general, the risk to the patient of an acute hemorrhage (e.g. gastrointestinal or intracranial bleed) far outweighs the risk of thrombosis on a metal valve and the warfarin should be reversed with fresh frozen plasma ± vitamin K until the hemorrhagic risk has subsided. Even the highest estimates of the risk of prosthetic valve thrombosis without any anticoagulation are around 30–50% per year (~0.5–1% per week). The short term bleeding risk in acute hemorrhage is usually much higher than this, so the balance of risks is in favor of treating the hemorrhage and accepting a small risk of valve thrombosis.

Elective procedures requiring cessation of anticoagulation
- Some procedures (e.g. dental extraction) can be done with a lowering of the INR to ~2.5 rather than cessation of warfarin
- For surgery or other procedures where anticoagulation needs stopping, heparin transition is not needed if patients have a bileaflet AVR and no additional risk factors for thromboembolism (i.e., AF, prior thromboembolism,

Box 9.7 (Continued)

hypercoagulable or severe LV dysfunction). All other patients undergoing elective surgery should preferably be admitted for a few days for unfractionated heparin; low molecular weight heparin is also acceptable as an outpatient while Coumadin is being held. Anticoagulation should resume postoperatively as soon as the bleeding risk is acceptably low as determined by the surgeon.

Acute Rheumatic Fever

This is an immunologically mediated systemic inflammatory illness, with a significant cardiac component, several weeks following group A streptococcal infection (often a sore throat). The incidence now is very low in developed world, but it is more common in the Indian sub-continent, the Middle East, and among Australian aboriginals. It commonly affects children age 5–15, but long-term damage to cardiac valves may result in problems in later life.

Presentation

Carditis

Regurgitant (especially a mitral) murmur is the most common clinical feature.

- Onset tends to be insidious
- A pan-carditis can occur, with pericarditis, myocarditis, and endocarditis:
  - Endocarditis, affecting the valves, is the most important aspect, and acute heart failure or chronic problems are usually due to this
  - Pericarditis ± effusion is common but rarely causes problems
  - Myocarditis may cause acute LV dysfunction, but this is rare
  - AV block (usually 1°)

Arthritis

- More rapid onset, over hours or days
- Large-joint, migratory polyarthritis (e.g. knees, ankles, wrists, elbows). It can be exquisitely painful—one joint tends to predominate.

Other

- Fever (common); abdominal pain (rare)
- Sydenham's chorea ('St. Vitus' dance')—rhythmic, involuntary upper limb movements. This is usually a prolonged latent period (6 months). It often resolves after 6 weeks but occasionally lasts up to 6 months; usually affects females

- Subcutaneous nodules and erythema marginatum.

→ Consider infective arthritis in any child with a fever and non-specific arthralgia.

Treatment

- The patient should be on bed rest until arthritis and any heart failure have resolved
- Penicillin for any remaining streptococci: penicillin G 1.2 MU single dose IM or penicillin V 250 mg po (adults 500 mg) tds for 10 days; give erythromycin if penicillin-allergic at a dose of 20–40 mg/kg/d (adults 250 mg qds)
- Aspirin or other NSAIDs for arthritis (usually high dose: 80–100 mg/kg/d; adults 4–8 g/d, in divided doses)
- Corticosteroids are often still used, but evidence for any benefit is low; if used, prescribe prednisolone 40–60 mg/d, tapering after 2–3 weeks
- Treat heart failure; consider valve replacement if there is severe dysfunction
- Prescribe haloperidol or other drugs for chorea.

Prevention of Recurrence

Secondary prophylaxis is required—penicillin V 250 mg bd (or IM penicillin G 1.2 MU every 3 weeks). The minimum duration is 5 years or until age 21 (whichever is later). However, if there is severe valve destruction, prophylaxis should continue to age 30 or more.

Table 9.4 Modified Jones Criteria for Diagnosis of Initial Attack of Acute Rheumatic Fever (1992)*

Diagnosis requires both:

Demonstration of current/recent group A streptococcal infection.
(culture or serological tests e.g. anti-streptolysin O. Chorea and late-onset carditis are exempt.)
And

2 major, or 1 major plus 2 minor criteria:

Major Criteria	Minor Criteria
• Carditis	• Fever
• Polyarthritis	• Arthralgia
• Chorea	• Elevated acute phase reactants
• Subcutaneous nodules	• Prolonged PR interval.
• Erythema marginatum.	

*Recurrent attacks require only 1 major or 2 minor criteria, plus evidence of recent Gp A streptococcus and no other explanation for symptoms.

Source: Guidelines for the diagnosis of rheumatic fever. Jones Criteria, 1992 update. *JAMA.* 1992; 268(15): 2069–73.

Affected valves

Mitral: 65–70%
Aortic: 25%
Tricuspid: 10%, with other valves often involved
Pulmonary: rare

Acute effects

Inflammation, destruction, and valve regurgitation.

Long term effects

(30–50%; 70% if severe carditis during acute phase):
- Regurgitation
- Stenosis due to scarring and contraction following the acute inflammation
- Valves typically appear thickened, with rolled edges and tips on echocardiography.

Valve repair

If valve surgery is required, valves might be suitable for repair during the acute episode, but are usually unsuitable for repair in the chronic stage.

Aortic Stenosis

This is the most common valve lesion; its prevalence is about 2% in those older than 65 years of age.

Causes

- Degenerative (most common)
- Bicuspid aortic valve (in which case there may be accelerated degeneration). Bicuspid valves also have an association with both coarctation and aortic dilatation ± dissection, even in the absence of aortic valve dysfunction
- Previous rheumatic fever.

Clinical Features

Symptoms

- There may be none
- SOB, syncope or angina may all occur and signify a poor prognosis.

Signs

- Harsh, musical, ejection systolic murmur best heard in the aortic region, radiating to carotids

- In severe stenosis there is a slow-rising pulse, a heaving non-displaced apex, and a soft or absent 2nd heart sound
- LV hypertrophy on the EKG.

Differential diagnosis: Consider sub-aortic obstruction, and hypertrophic obstructive cardiomyopathy.

Acute Problems

Acute Presentation of Chronic Disease

- Symptom onset can be rapid (days or weeks) and should prompt consideration for aortic valve replacement (AVR)
- If LV function is poor, there may be in intractable pulmonary edema and aortic valve replacement is the only treatment. Many patients improve if they survive surgery.

Acute stenosis

- Rare
- Causes: thrombus on prosthetic valve, vegetation
- Usually requires prompt aortic valve replacement.

Treatment

Aortic valve replacement

This is the only real cure and is performed if there is symptomatic severe aortic stenosis.

Medical (for temporary relief)

- Dyspnea can be treated with diuretics
- Beta-blockers may be useful, particularly for angina
- Vasodilator drugs should be used cautiously.

Balloon valvuloplasty

This may be used in younger patients (who have a less calcified valve) as a holding measure to defer surgery (e.g. if pregnant).

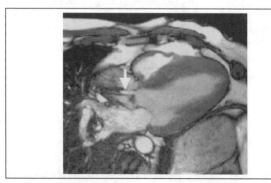

Figure 9.6 Cardiac magnetic resonance image of severe aortic stenosis, demonstrating a high velocity eccentric jet of aortic flow.

Aortic Regurgitation

Causes

Acute: Type A aortic dissection, aortic valve endocarditis, and trauma.

Chronic: Previous infective endocarditis, aortic root dilatation (including Marfan syndrome), degenerative valve, and previous rheumatic fever.

Clinical Features

- Acute aortic regurgitation causes sudden severe shortness of breath and pulmonary edema
- In severe chronic disease, shortness of breath may be the only symptom.

Signs

- Early diastolic, decrescendo murmur heard at the lower left sternal edge, best heard in expiration
- ± Ejection systolic flow murmur (increased forward flow across valve)
- In severe disease:
  - Collapsing pulse
  - Displaced, hyperdynamic apex (due to dilated LV)
  - Other eponymous signs, mostly due to widened pulse pressure (see Table 9.5).

Acute Problems

Acute (sudden) regurgitation

- The patient is extremely unwell, often in pulmonary edema
- Needs emergency valve replacement (± aortic root replacement if there is dissection)
- Holding treatments while surgery is being arranged: diuretics, vasodilators, inotropes, ventilation. Do not place on an intra-aortic balloon pump as this worsens the regurgitation.

Acute presentation of chronic disease

Once symptoms develop in chronic disease, aortic valve replacement should be considered.

Mixed Aortic Valve Disease

- *Causes:* Bicuspid valve, rheumatic heart disease, endocarditis on aortic stenosis, previous (partially successful) valvuloplasty for stenosis

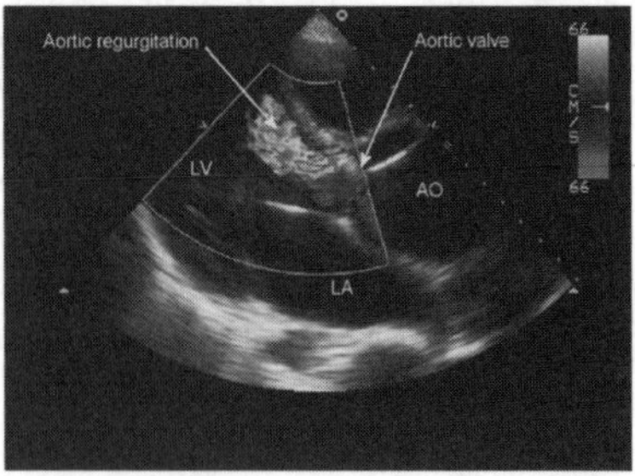

Figure 9.7 Parasternal transthoracic echocardiogram demonstrating a broad jet of aortic regurgitation in a patient with a dilated aorta (AO).

Table 9.5 Eponymous Signs in Severe AR	
Sign	**Clinical Features**
Corrigan's	Visible carotid pulsation.
de Musset's	Head bobbing with each pulse.
Müller's	Visible uvula pulsation.
Quincke's	Visible capillary pulsation in nailbed.
Traube's	Systolic & diastolic femoral sounds ('pistol-shot' femorals).
Duroziez's	Compression of femoral artery proximally causes systolic bruit; distal compression causes proximal bruit.

- True mixed aortic valve disease should be differentiated from aortic regurgitation with increased systolic aortic flow velocity secondary to increased stroke volume, and from aortic stenosis with a mild leak
- The relative severity of each component (stenosis and regurgitation) is variable, though predominant stenosis is more common and is the more significant problem
- The combination of a narrowed outlet and the need for increased stroke volume places substantial demands on the myocardium, and the LV is often very hypertrophied and responds poorly to rapid changes. Acute problems can therefore occur more readily, e.g. deterioration with the onset of AF.

Mitral Stenosis

Incidence has significantly declined in developed countries due to the reduction in its major cause: rheumatic fever.

Causes

- Previous rheumatic fever
- Other rare causes: congenital, bulky vegetation, atrial myxoma.

Clinical Features

Acute mitral stenosis is extraordinarily rare. Most present chronically with an insidious onset of dyspnea, fatigue or reduced exercise tolerance.

Signs: Atrial fibrillation is common. Look for a malar flush and prominent 'a' waves in the JVP.

Auscultation: Listen for a prominent S1, opening snap, low-pitched mid-diastolic rumbling murmur with pre-systolic accentuation (from atrial contraction).

EKG: Bifid P wave (± peaked P wave if pulmonary HT), AF.

Acute Problems

- Often caused by an increased heart rate. This is tolerated badly due to the increased time required for passage of blood across the stenotic valve
- Common causes: AF, exercise, infection (esp. chest), pregnancy
- Present with SOB ± heart failure.

Atrial fibrillation

With acute AF, the loss of atrial contraction in addition to the sudden increase in heart rate can rapidly precipitate heart failure.

Treatment

The combination of heart failure and moderate to severe mitral stenosis is difficult to treat. An urgent cardiology consultation should be sought immediately.

- Diuretics
- Rate control (digoxin for AF; diltiazem/verapamil, beta-blockers)—this is a difficult balance in a patient with heart failure
- Consider cardioversion for acute AF (although this is not useful for chronic AF)
- Consider a balloon valvuloplasty.

Longer Term Issues

Atrial fibrillation

Permanent AF is common in mitral stenosis and rate control is required.

→ Anticoagulation is vital—thrombotic risk is huge (at least eleven times the risk compared with other causes of AF).

Surgery should be arranged for those with symptoms or pulmonary hypertension. Options are:

- Closed valvotomy (separation of fused cusps)
- Open valvotomy (on cardiac bypass)
- Mitral valve replacement.

Balloon valvuloplasty

- For valves without significant calcification or regurgitation
- Can give moderate relief for several months/years but restenosis usually occurs
- Particularly good for acute presentations in pregnancy.

Mitral Regurgitation

Causes

The mitral valve is a complex structure, relying on the papillary muscles, chordae and myocardial motion for its effective function. Intrinsic valve disease may not therefore be the only cause of dysfunction, and other reasons should be excluded.

Acute: Infective endocarditis, MI (papillary muscle infarction, rupture, or tethering to infarcted LV wall), ruptured chordae tendinae, trauma.

Chronic: Degenerative disease, mitral prolapse, dilated LV, myocardial dysfunction due to ischemia, and previous rheumatic fever.

Clinical Features

Symptoms

- Acute MR causes sudden, severe SOB and pulmonary edema
- Chronic disease may be asymptomatic for many years
- In severe chronic disease, SOB may be the only symptom and should prompt consideration of valve replacement.

Signs

- Pan-systolic murmur (soft, blowing) at apex, radiating to axilla
- If severe:
  - Wide splitting of S2, due to early aortic valve closure
  - Loud S3
  - Displaced, hyperdynamic apex.

Acute Problems

Acute (sudden) regurgitation

- Most common cause is post-MI (papillary muscle involvement)
- Patient is extremely unwell, and often in pulmonary edema
- Needs emergency valve replacement or repair of papillary muscle
- Holding treatments while surgery is arranged: diuretics, inotropes, vasodilators, ventilation, intra-aortic balloon pump.

Acute presentation of chronic disease

Like aortic regurgitation, once symptoms develop in chronic disease, valve replacement or repair should be considered, but it is important to exclude a 'functional' cause for MR such as a dilated LV with poor function, or ischemia, as these should be treated directly.

In chronic MR, left ventricular pressure is off-loaded by the flow of blood into the low pressure left atrium. Therefore the function should appear good and, in severe MR, even vigorous. A normal or slightly reduced ejection fraction in the presence of severe MR may thus in fact represent early LV dysfunction. Systolic LV dilation on echocardiography (>4.5 cm) is a good indicator of LV dysfunction.

Box 9.9 Mitral Prolapse (floppy mitral valve)

- Mostly idiopathic, prevalence 5–10% of the population
- If no or trivial regurgitation is present, it does not need follow up
- ≥ mild regurgitation needs follow-up and endocarditis prophylaxis
- Symptoms are from ectopic beats. Reports of atypical chest pain are inconsistent
- There is a classical late-systolic murmur if regurgitation is present
- Can degenerate to severe mitral regurgitation requiring surgery.

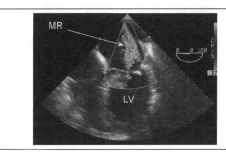

Figure 9.8 Transesophageal echocardiogram demonstrating mitral regurgitation.

Box 9.10 Surgery in Mitral Regurgitation

Valve replacement

This should be considered for intrinsic, severe disease unsuitable for repair. Metal prostheses are used—bioprosthetic valves tend to degenerate quickly, and are not routinely placed in the mitral position.

Box 9.10 (Continued)

Valve repair

This is ideal for severe MR where the valve anatomy is otherwise reasonably normal, such as in mitral valve prolapse. Rheumatic and other damaged valves are not usually suitable. Posterior leaflet repair is much more successful than anterior, though it is a technically demanding operation and both types require an experienced surgeon. Even in the best hands, repair is not always successful, and replacement is the fall-back position. Long term results are good in selected cases, and minimally-invasive repair, utilizing robotic arms, has been successful in a handful of cases to date.

Valve ring insertion

For cases where the mitral annulus is enlarged, causing failure of coaptation of the leaflets (either LV or LA enlargement). A 'C' shaped ring is sewn around the valve to reduce the annular size and restore integrity of function. Commonly combined with valve repair for prolapse with dilated LA/LV and with CABG for ischemic, dilated LV and functional regurgitation.

Papillary muscle repair

In cases of papillary rupture (usually secondary to MI), re-attachment of the papillary muscle may be all that is required for restoration of valve function. CABG may be performed at the same time, to deal with the coronary stenosis, but this depends on the clinical situation.

Pulmonary Stenosis

Causes

Congenital (may be in conjunction with other defects, e.g. Fallot's tetralogy), rheumatic fever, carcinoid.

Clinical Features

There are few symptoms—SOB if severe.
Signs: RV heave, prominent a wave in JVP ± tricuspid regurgitation, quiet P2, soft ejection systolic murmur at upper left sternal edge.
EKG: RVH, P pulmonale.

Acute Problems

These are rare, but a rapid increase in heart rate can lead to right-sided heart failure.

Treatment

- Balloon valvuloplasty is the usual first-line treatment. It is effective and may be repeated in future. Pulmonary regurgitation is the main side effect and is usually tolerated well

- Surgical (open) valvotomy is also very effective with good long term results
- Pulmonary valve replacement (rarely required).

Pulmonary Regurgitation

Causes
Congenital, endocarditis, secondary to pulmonary hypertension, following balloon valvuloplasty or open valvotomy.

Clinical Features
Pulmonary regurgitation is usually tolerated extremely well. These will be SOB if it is very severe, and RV failure occurs.
Signs: RV heave, loud ± delayed P2, ± soft pulmonary ejection murmur, diastolic decrescendo murmur at mid left sternal edge, RV failure.
EKG: RVH.

Acute Problems
These are rare. Right ventricular failure may develop and present acutely; acute pulmonary hypertension (e.g. from pulmonary embolus) may cause pulmonary regurgitation.

Treatment
- Usually none required, because it is tolerated very well
- Treat any RV failure
- Treat the cause of pulmonary hypertension
- If there are severe symptoms and RV failure, pulmonary valve replacement can be considered
- New techniques include a bioprosthetic valve mounted on a stent, which can be inserted percutaneously.

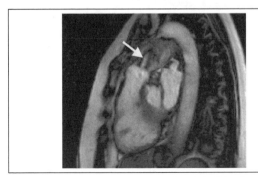

Figure 9.9 Cardiac magnetic resonance image showing the RV outflow tract. There is significant pulmonary stenosis (arrow indicates high velocity jet).

Tricuspid Stenosis

Causes

Rheumatic fever (usually in association with mitral stenosis), carcinoid, very rarely with a pacemaker lead.

Clinical Features

The main and often only feature is fatigue.

Signs: Raised JVP with prominent 'a' wave, mid-diastolic murmur at left sternal edge—similar to mitral stenosis but higher pitch, hepatomegaly and peripheral edema if severe.

Acute Problems

- Almost never
- Acute stenosis could occur with large infective vegetation.

Treatment

- Diuretics
- Balloon valvuloplasty or surgical valvotomy at the time other (usually mitral) lesions are dealt with
- Valve replacement is avoided due to the difficulty with low right-sided venous pressures and the resistance to flow from a prosthetic valve.

Tricuspid Regurgitation

Causes

Congenital (including Ebstein's anomaly), Marfan, any cause of RV dilatation, pulmonary hypertension, endocarditis and carcinoid.

Clinical Features

- Minimal symptoms
- Right heart failure can develop if severe
- *Signs:* Large 'v' waves in JVP, pulsatile hepatomegaly, (peripheral edema, ascites ± jaundice if significant RV failure), very soft pansystolic murmur at left sternal edge.

Acute Problems

- Rare
- Tricuspid endocarditis may occur in IV drug users, and is usually staphylococcal. It follows an aggressive course and needs intensive antibiotic treatment.

Treatment

- Usually none required
- Diuretics are the mainstay of treatment for symptoms and RV failure
- Tricuspid valvuloplasty, annuloplasty, and valve replacement are rarely undertaken and long term results are disappointing.

Chapter 10

Aortic Dissection

Aortic Dissection

An aortic dissection is a tear in the aortic intima through which blood enters the aortic wall and strips the media from the adventitia.

- The dissection may result in fatal aortic rupture or propagate distally generating a blood-filled space between the dissected layers
- The blood supply to major branches (including the coronary arteries) may be compromised
- If the aortic root is involved, the aortic valve may become incompetent and retrograde propagation to the pericardium may result in cardiac tamponade.

The most common site for aortic dissection is in the *proximal ascending aorta* within a few centimeters of the aortic valve or in the descending aorta just distal to the left subclavian artery.

Classification is usually made according to the Stanford classification that influences subsequent management:

Type A aortic dissection involves the ascending aorta and management is a surgical emergency. Move quickly.

Type B aortic dissection spares the ascending aorta and its management is initially medical, with urgent blood pressure control and pain relief.

Causes and Associations

- Hypertension (70%)
- Bicuspid aortic valve (7–14%) (see p. 133)
- Marfan syndrome (5–9%) (see p. 149)
- Aortic coarctation (see p. 189)
- Iatrogenic (angiography).

Presentation

The cardinal symptom is *pain* and is usually instantaneous, of cataclysmic severity, pulsatile or tearing, in the anterior thorax or interscapular region, and migrates as the dissection propagates. However, dissection pain can be quite varied, so if you don't think about it you won't find it.

Clinical Signs

Remember that the classical signs may not be present.

- The patient may appear shocked but blood pressure can be normal or elevated
- Pulmonary edema can occur due to severe aortic regurgitation
- Absent or reduced pulses occur in 20% of patients (but can fluctuate)
- Signs of aortic regurgitation or pericardial tamponade can occur in Type A aortic dissection
- A left pleural effusion is occasionally seen on chest X-ray.

Investigations

CXR

- An abnormal aortic silhouette appears in up to 90% of cases. However, at least 10% of chest X-rays will appear normal
- Separation of the intimal calcification that occurs in the aortic knob by more than 1 cm (the 'calcium sign') is suggestive of aortic dissection
- Left-sided pleural effusions can occur and are more common with descending dissections.

EKG

- Non-specific ST and T wave changes are common
- EKG changes of left ventricular hypertrophy may occur in patients with long-standing hypertension, but this is hardly a diagnostic finding
- Although coronary artery involvement is uncommon when it does occur, it more commonly affects the right coronary artery, resulting in inferior ST elevation.

Blood tests

There is no role for blood tests in making the diagnosis.
Do not wait for any results before arranging further imaging or intervention.

Imaging

Computed tomography

With modern spiral scanners, this has a sensitivity and specificity of 96–100% and is the standard investigation for suspected aortic dissection.

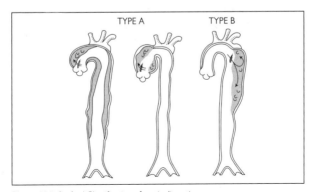

Figure 10.1 Sanford Classification of aortic dissection.
Type A: All dissections involving the ascending aorta. Type B dissection does not involve the ascending aorta.

Magnetic resonance imaging

MRI has a sensitivity and specificity of nearly 100%, and is non-invasive. However, its limited availability and the difficulty in placing an unstable patient in the scanner limits its use.

Transesophageal echocardiography

This is useful for imaging the proximal ascending aorta, identifying involvement of coronary ostia, and examining the aortic valve. It has a sensitivity of >98% and specificity of ~95%. Patients usually require sedation. It is ideally performed immediately prior to surgery after surgical consent has been obtained.

Transthoracic echocardiography

Can determine the involvement of the aortic valve, left ventricular function and identify pericardial effusions. It is far less of a good test, with a sensitivity of 59–85% and specificity of 63–96%. Hence, a normal transthoracic echocardiogram does not exclude aortic dissection.

Aortography

This is an invasive procedure with associated risks. It requires contrast material and takes time to perform. Since the advent of CT it is now rarely performed as other imaging techniques are quicker and safer.

Coronary angiography

Not routinely performed in patients with aortic dissection. Chronic coronary disease is seen in a quarter of patients with aortic dissection but this has not been shown to have a significant impact on outcome.

Differential Diagnosis

- Intramural hematoma (see p. 150)
- Penetrating atherosclerotic ulcer (see p. 150)
- Acute coronary syndrome (see p. 42)

Pharmacological Management

- Opiate analgesia should be given to eliminate pain (e.g. morphine sulfate 4 mg IV, q15 minutes prn)
- Lower systolic blood pressure to less than 120 mmHg with intravenous antihypertensive drugs:
  - Beta-blockers and the vasodilator sodium nitroprusside are the traditional first-line therapies (see Box 10.1)
  - IV isosorbide dinitrate and oral nifedipine are alternatives in patients with contraindications to beta-blockers.

In hypotensive patients, it is important to exclude pericardial tamponade and check the blood pressure in both arms before commencing fluid resuscitation. Pericardiocentesis should not be performed prior to surgery, as it can precipitate irretrievable hemodynamic collapse.

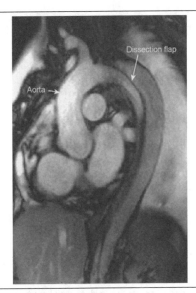

Figure 10.2 Magnetic resonance image of a Type B aortic dissection.
There is a dissection flap in the descending aorta.

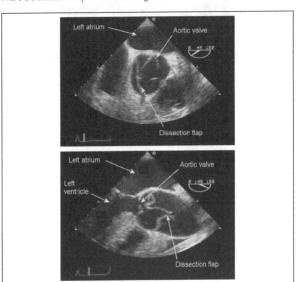

Figure 10.3 Transesophageal echocardiography showing a Type A aortic dissection.
Just above the aortic valve in the proximal ascending aorta is a dissection flap.
Top: transverse view. Bottom: longitudinal view.

Box 10.1 Intravenous Antihypertensive Therapy

- Labetalol is a beta-blocker with alpha-blocking effects at high doses. It is given as an intravenous injection of 50 mg over 1 minute followed by a continuous infusion of 1–2 mg/min
- Esmolol is a short-acting beta-blocker. It is administered as a bolus of 500 mcg/kg and as an infusion of 50–200 mcg/kg/min
- Propranolol is given as an intravenous injection of 1 mg over 1 minute and repeated every 5 minutes until an adequate response has been achieved or a total of 10 mg has been given. Additional propranolol should then be given every 4 hours
- Sodium nitroprusside is given as an initial infusion of 0.5–1.5 mcg/kg/min, increasing in steps of 0.5 mcg/kg/min every 5 minutes. Dose range 0.5–8 mcg/kg/min. It is usually given with a beta-blocker to prevent reflex tachycardia.

Surgical Management

Type A aortic dissection (involving the ascending aorta) should be treated with emergency surgical repair.

Type B aortic dissections are usually managed medically. Surgery for type B dissections should be considered if there is evidence of proximal extension, progressive aortic enlargement, or ischemic complications from major branch artery involvement.

Endovascular Aortic Stenting

Endovascular stenting is a percutaneous procedure that may be considered for aortic dissection starting distal to the left subclavian artery or to treat the complications of penetrating aortic ulcers.

Complications of Aortic Dissection

Type A
- Death from aortic rupture
- Myocardial ischemia/infarction
- Pericardial tamponade
- Aortic valve incompetence
- Cerebrovascular event.

Type B
- Visceral ischemia
- Limb ischemia
- Renal failure.

Prognosis

- The mortality from aortic dissection is initially as high as 1% per hour
- The surgical mortality is about 10–15% for type A dissection and slightly higher for type B
- The long-term survival for patients with either surgically treated type A or medically treated type B dissections is about 75% at 5 years.

Follow up

- Long-term oral antihypertensive therapy should be initiated to maintain a systolic blood pressure below 130 mmHg
- Drug therapies include beta-blockers, ACE-inhibitors, and calcium antagonists
- Surveillance is recommended for all patients using the imaging modality with which there is the most local expertise, particularly in the first two years after presentation
- Surgery or endovascular stenting should be considered if there is evidence of progressive aortic enlargement.

Marfan Syndrome

- Autosomal dominant connective tissue disease with a prevalence of at least 1:10,000
- Common cardiovascular features are:
  - mitral valve prolapse (75%)
  - dilatation of the aortic sinuses (90%)
- Aortic dilatation is usually limited to the proximal ascending aorta with loss of the sinotubular junction and a flask-shape appearance
- Aortic regurgitation is common when the aorta reaches 50 mm in diameter (normal diameter <40 mm)
- The risk of dissection increases with the diameter of the aorta but occurs relatively infrequently below a diameter of 55 mm
- Aortic dissection in Marfan syndrome is usually Type A and begins just above the coronary ostia. 10% of cases begin distal to the left subclavian artery (Type B)
- Beta blockade has been shown to reduce the rate of aortic dilatation and reduce the risk of aortic dissection
- Surgery is usually considered when the aorta reaches >50 mm.

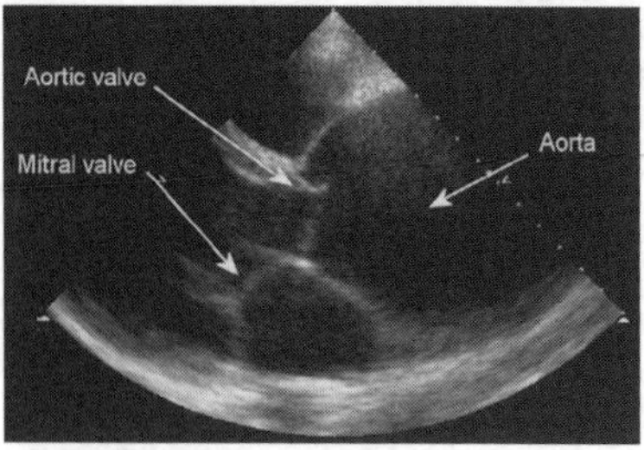

Figure 10.4 Transthoracic echocardiography of an enlarged ascending aorta in a patient with Marfan syndrome.

Acute Thoracic Syndromes

These syndromes may mimic acute aortic dissection.

Intramural Hematoma

- The result of hemorrhage within the media and adventitia of the aortic wall. The aortic intima remains intact
- Believed to be due to rupture of the aortic vasa vasorum
- Presentation can mimic aortic dissection
- Patients are typically elderly, with a history of hypertension and many have aortic atherosclerosis
- The diagnosis is made by excluding an intimal tear
- Computed tomography and magnetic resonance imaging are the investigations of choice. A non-contrast-enhancing crescent along the aortic wall with no false lumen or associated atherosclerotic ulcer is usually demonstrated
- There is increasing evidence that an intramural hematoma may be a precursor of aortic dissection
- Treat as for aortic dissection with IV analgesia and anti-hypertensive agents
- Surgery is indicated when the ascending aorta is involved.

Penetrating Atherosclerotic Ulcer

- Ulceration of an atherosclerotic lesion of the aorta that penetrates the elastic lamina of the aorta allowing hematoma formation within the media
- Usually in the descending aorta in elderly smokers
- Clinical presentation is similar to aortic dissection with chest or back pain

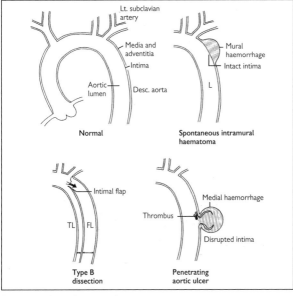

Figure 10.5 Acute thoracic syndromes.
An intramural hematoma is characterized by an intact intima. Type B aortic dissection usually starts distal to the left subclavian artery. A penetrating aortic ulcer involves a disrupted intima and hemorrhage into the media.

- In up to 25% of cases, penetration through to the adventitia results in false aneurysm formation and transmural aortic rupture occurs in up to 10% of cases
- Aortography is the diagnostic standard
- The standard treatment is surgery but there has been increasing success with the use of endovascular stenting.

Chapter 11

Pericardial Disease

Pericarditis

Acute inflammation of the pericardium characteristically produces chest pain, low-grade fever and a pericardial friction rub. Pericarditis and myocarditis commonly coexist.

History

The usual presentation is of sharp chest pain which is worse on inspiration or movement. Many patients will describe relief when sitting forward. Chest pain is typically sharp, central, and retrosternal. A pericardial effusion may cause dysphagia by compressing the esophagus. There may be a low-grade fever and a history of a recent viral infection.

Physical Exam

Classical features of acute pericarditis are a friction rub and concordant ST elevation on EKG. The rub is best heard over the lower left sternal edge with the patient sitting forward. The characteristic combination of clinical presentation and EKG changes often allows a definite diagnosis.

A pericardial friction rub is often intermittent, positional, and elusive. It tends to be louder during inspiration and may be heard in both systole and diastole. Low-grade fever is common. Rarely, with a very large effusion, signs of tamponade may be present. Look for Kussmaul's sign, which is the inspiratory distention of the neck veins (the opposite of the normally seen expiratory distention). It is a sign of constrictive pericarditis (as well as right-sided CHF), and caused by impaired right heart filling during the negative intrathoracic pressure generated by inspiration.

Investigation

The EKG is the first step of the essential investigation. Look for diffuse ST segment elevation with the ST segments being concave up. In later stages of pericarditis the ST elevation resolves and there may be flattened or inverted T waves and a flattened PR segment.

The EKG changes result from associated epicardial inflammation. Sinus tachycardia is usual, but atrial fibrillation or flutter as well as ectopic beats may occur. The ST elevation is concave up (in contrast to MI—see p. 48) and present in at least 2 limb leads and all chest leads (most marked in V_{3-6}). T waves are initially prominent, upright, and peaked, becoming flattened or inverted over several days. PR depression (reflecting atrial inflammation) may occur in the same leads as ST elevation (this PR-ST discordance is characteristic). Pathological Q waves do not develop at any stage. A pericardial effusion causes decreased QRS amplitude in all leads. Very occasionally, electrical alternans is also seen (and is diagnostic).

Appropriate investigations include an EKG, CBC, and BMP. An ESR is used to follow response to therapy, but will not help in making the initial diagnosis. If the patient is anticoagulated, check the INR, since hemorrhage may cause pericarditis. Cardiac troponins are not a discriminator between MI and pericarditis.

An echocardiogram is rarely needed, but should be considered in patients with pericarditis who are systemically unwell or hypotensive. It can also be useful to exclude acute MI in difficult cases. (The ECHO should demonstrate regional left ventricular dysfunction corresponding to coronary artery territory in an MI.)

It is also unusual to need to aspirate the pericardial effusion, but if fluid is obtained send it to the lab for Ziehl-Nielsen staining, cytology, protein, LDH (see p. 254 for the technique of pericardiocentesis).

Radiological Studies

A plain chest X-ray is not usually helpful. However, an enlarged cardiac silhouette suggests a significant effusion and should be followed by echocardiography, which is the test of choice when a pericardial effusion is suspected. Clinical evidence of cardiac tamponade is rare, and there is no need to obtain an urgent Echo in all patients with a diagnosis of pericarditis. However, if patients have the following features, an urgent bedside ED Echo is required:

Ill appearing   Muffled heart sounds
Dyspnea   Elevated JVD
Hypotension

Intervention

Most patients with idiopathic or post-viral pericarditis may be treated with NSAIDs and discharged. In cases of cardiac tamponade (see p. 156) due to pericarditis, a fluid bolus of 1–2 liters should be administered. Pericardiocentesis (see p. 254) is required in order to drain the pericardial sac and restore normal cardiac output, and should be performed in the ED if the patient has any signs of tamponade.

Causes

There are several different etiologies that need be considered in a patient with pericarditis:

- Idiopathic causes are common
- Viral (e.g. coxsackie B virus, HIV)—the most common cause
- Myocardial infarction (including Dressler's syndrome—see below)
- Bacterial (pneumonia and/or septicemia)
- TB (especially in patients with HIV)
- Locally invasive carcinoma (e.g. bronchus or breast)
- Rheumatic fever—see p. 131
- Uremia

- Collagen vascular disease (SLE, polyarteritis nodosa, rheumatoid arthritis)
- Hypothyroidism
- After cardiac surgery or radiotherapy
- Trauma (e.g. blunt chest injury see p. 239).

Consultation

Patients with significant findings on physical exam or by echo should be referred to cardiology or cardiothoracic surgery (who may open a pericardial window).

Disposition and Documentation

In most cases, viral pericarditis is usually benign and self-limiting, responding to symptomatic treatment (rest and NSAIDs). Document a normal physical exam and results of any investigations, as well as close follow-up and instructions to return for worse pain or trouble breathing. If your investigation reveals a cause (such as uremic pericarditis), your interventions should be noted.

Differentiating Pericarditis from Acute Ischemia

This is usually straightforward, but there are more difficult cases. Focus on the history, especially the character of pain. Patients with pericarditis are younger and usually relatively well compared to typical MI patients, and should not be diaphoretic, clammy, or appear pale or grey.

The EKG can sometimes look like an acute MI but does not have reciprocal changes, and the history and well appearance of the patient are usually clues against this. The correct diagnosis is important, as giving thrombolysis to a patient with pericarditis can risk hemorrhagic tamponade. If in real doubt, an echocardiogram can be helpful.

Pericardial Tamponade

Tamponade occurs when the heart is unable to contract normally due to fluid accumulation in the pericardial sac. Only 100–200 cc of fluid is needed to impair cardiac filing and rapidly decrease cardiac output.

History

The classic history is of pleuritic chest pain, shortness of breath, cough, and fatigue. Ask about recent viral syndromes that may be associated with pericarditis. Ask also about underlying malignancy. Penetrating chest trauma may cause tamponade; suspect it if there is hypotension, tachycardia and an elevated JVP, but remember first to look for and treat any pneumothorax. Finally remember that a bacterial infection may lead to an infectious effusion resulting rarely in tamponade.

Physical Exam

There is usually hypotension. The heart sounds are muffled, and there may be a pericardial friction rub. The rub is best heard over the lower left sternal edge with the patient sitting forward. The JVD is elevated and the liver is often engorged. Measure the BP and look for pulsus paradoxus, a decrease in the pulse volume during inspiration, which results in an abnormally decreased BP (~12 mmHg) during inspiration. Beck's triad of hypotension, elevated JVP, and muffled heart sounds is only seen in about a third of all patients; finding all three signs is a late manifestation of tamponade and suggests that cardiac arrest is impending.

Investigation

The EKG will show a low voltage electrical alterans.

Radiological Studies

In cases of chronic effusions leading to slowly worsening tamponade, the CXR will show an enlarged cardiac silhouette. However, this will more commonly be from cardiomegaly. The imaging modality of choice is bedside echocardiography. In tamponade there is a circumferential effusion with a hyperdynamic heart that shows diastolic right ventricular or right atrial collapse. Other findings on ECHO include:

- Diastolic collapse of right ventricular free wall and right atrium
- Dilated inferior vena cava with no inspiratory collapse and reversed flow with atrial contraction
- Increased tricuspid flow during inspiration
- Decreased mitral flow during inspiration.

Intervention

If tamponade is suspected, place the patient in the resuscitation suite and start two large-bore IVs. If the patient is unstable or does not respond to IV fluids perform an ED pericardiocentesis (see p. 254). Traumatic tamponade requires an emergent thoracotomy. Be prepared to perform a pericardiocentesis to stabilize the patient until this can be arranged. Removing only a small amount of fluid can considerably improve the hemodynamic situation. If a patient in the emergency department with a traumatic tamponade loses his vital signs, perform a thoracotomy.

Differential Diagnosis

There are several other clinical entities which may present with one or more findings suggestive of tamponade. Make sure you have addressed each before diagnosing tamponade.

CHF	Sepsis
PE	Aortic dissection
Tension pneumothorax	

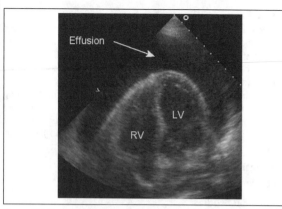

Figure 11.1 Transthoracic echocardiography demonstrating a large pericardial effusion over-lying the left (LV) and right (RV) ventricles.

Consultation

For all cases of traumatic tamponade, call for a stat ED consult from the trauma or general surgeon. In stable medical cases, consult with cardiology to ascertain which interventions they may prefer.

Disposition and Documentation

All cases of tamponade are admitted to the ICU. Document carefully the timing of your interventions, as well as the reasoning behind any decision to delay intervention.

Constrictive Pericarditis

Constrictive pericarditis resembles congestive cardiac failure but the clinical picture is not due to failure, rather the cardiac function has been impeded due to impaired filling.

History

Most cases are idiopathic. The initial acute episode may be subclinical, and result from viral, tuberculous, and pyogenic infections. Ask about obvious known causes like therapeutic irradiation or recent cardiac surgery.

Physical Exam

Look for chronic venous congestion and an elevated JVP. (The classic prominent *x* and *y* descents of the JVP wave are difficult to see). Check for ankle and sacral edema, and abdominal distension. There may be ascites and hepatosplenomegaly. The heart sounds often reveal a loud or palpable S_3 due to the blood rapidly entering the stiff ventricle, known as a pericardial knock. There may be hypotension in severe cases and atrial arrhythmias are common.

Investigations

The EKG usually shows non-specific T wave abnormalities with low voltages and broad P waves. Atrial fibrillation may be seen. The CXR findings that support the diagnosis are a pleural effusion and pericardial calcifications (the latter are best seen on the lateral films).

Echocardiography should be performed. Look for the following findings:

- Pericardial thickening and calcification with biatrial enlargement
- Rapid early filling (increased E:A ratio)
- Dilated vena cava and hepatic veins with restricted respiratory fluctuations
- Paradoxical ventricular septal movement with a flat posterior wall
- Increased tricuspid flow and reduced mitral flow in inspiration (similar to tamponade)

CT or MRI will show pericardial thickening (>6 mm) and calcifications, biatrial enlargement, and a dilated vena cava and hepatic veins.

Cardiac catheterization might be needed to differentiate the disease from restrictive cardiomyopathy (see p. 71) and to exclude co-existent coronary artery disease. Typical findings are:

- Left ventricular end diastolic pressure = right ventricular end diastolic pressure throughout respiration (in patients with a restrictive cardiomyopathy they usually differ by >7 mmHg). Both are elevated and have a dip and plateau (square root) configuration
- Atrial pressures are high and equal with prominent x and y descents.

Finally, remember to exclude TB, performing a tuberculin skin test and by sending at least three sputum samples.

Intervention and Management

A surgical pericardectomy is usually required, so consult early with the cardio-thoracic surgeons. Balloon dilatation of the pericardium can be considered as a palliative procedure. Start the patient on diuretic therapy and a salt-restricted diet.

Chapter 12

Pulmonary Vascular Disease

Pulmonary Embolus

Pulmonary embolism (PE) is a common life-threatening problem, responsible for many deaths each year. Unless you think about it you will not diagnose it. There may be no clinical evidence of DVT, and a PE will only be found in about one patient in twenty in whom you suspect the disease.

History

PE is notoriously difficult to diagnose. Suspect it in any patient with the classical signs of pleuritic chest pain, dyspnea, syncope, cough, or hemoptysis. About 75% of patients *with a proven PE* have one or more of the following risk factors:

- Prior PE
- DVT
- Recent immobilization
- Stroke
- Recent pregnancy
- Use of oral contraceptive pills
- Recent surgery
- Underlying malignancy

However, these figures mean that up to a quarter of all patients will have not one of these risk factors at presentation.

Physical Exam

The most common finding is tachypnea (85%). Look for signs of a DVT as well as right heart dysfunction (e.g. a loud pulmonary component of S2, a right-sided heave, or an S3). Not one of the signs or symptoms of a PE are pathognomonic, and many are neither sensitive nor specific:

Table 12.1 Symptoms in Patients with Proven PE (%)

Dyspnea	84	Hemoptysis	30
Pleuritic chest pain	74	Syncope	30
Apprehension	60	Sweating	25
Cough	50	Non-pleuritic chest pain	15

Table 12.2 Findings in Patients with Proven PE

Tachypnea	90%	Gallop	30%
Rales	60%	Peripheral edema	25%
Loud S2	55%	Heart murmur	20%
Tachycardia	45%	Cyanosis	15%
Diaphoresis	35%		

In a small PE, physical signs may be absent or subtle (mild fever, tachycardia, scattered crepitations or pleural rub). Search carefully for DVT.

In a large PE, the patient is usually cyanosed, tachycardic, dyspneic, and hypotensive. Turbulent flow around the PE occasionally produces an audible murmur in the pulmonary area.

Investigation

Most tests are as unreliable as the physical exam in helping you to diagnose a PE:

1. *CXR* Most patients with a PE have an abnormal chest X-ray, but the findings are often non-specific. Changes due to a PE include pulmonary oligemia (regional vascular paucity), an elevated hemidiaphragm, a small pleural effusion, or linear opacities. It is not possible to diagnose a PE from a CXR, but it is possible to exclude other diagnoses, like pneumonia. A CXR is also needed if a V/Q scan is ordered. Therefore, obtain a good quality CXR, not to help you make the diagnosis, but rather to help you exclude other pathologies. So if you see no obvious abnormalities on the CXR and you suspect a PE, do not be surprised.

2. *ABG* There is no reason to obtain an ABG in patients with a suspected PE. It is a painful and entirely unhelpful test because a large proportion of patients with a proven PE have a normal ABG.

3. *EKG* The classic finding of an $S_1Q_3T_3$ pattern is rarely seen (an S wave in I and a Q wave and inverted T wave in III). The most common changes are a sinus tachycardia, atrial fibrillation, RBBB, and right axis deviation (S_1). About 10% of patients with a PE have a completely normal EKG.

4. *Routine blood tests* A CBC and BMP cannot aid you in making the diagnosis. However, if these tests are routinely needed in order to admit a patient from the ED, it may be prudent to obtain them early in your evaluation.

5. *D-dimer* When fibrin is broken down, one of the degradation products is D-dimer. There are five major tests for D-dimer. The ELISA -dimer assay has a sensitivity for the diagnosis of PE of 97% and a specificity of 44%. Latex kits are rapid, but are not sensitive enough to reliably exclude PE. If the D-dimer is negative and you have a low clinical suspicion for a PE, there is good data that this is sufficient for you to rule out the diagnosis of PE. If, however, your pre-test probability is high, you should proceed to imaging and not rely on the D-dimer alone.

Radiological Studies

PE cannot be diagnosed on the basis of a plain chest X-ray. However, you should obtain one if you are going to get a V/Q scan, since it is needed in order to interpret the scan. A V/Q scan used to be widely used in order to diagnose a PE, but it needs to be interpreted in the setting of the clinical suspicion. This test may still be useful in some settings (e.g. a patient with dye allergy or renal failure), but a better test is a pulmonary angiogram performed by CT. This CT angiogram (CTA) is fast and very sensitive, although it also relies on the experience of the radiologist reading the images. The CTA is now the test of choice to diagnose a PE.

Bedside echocardiography is a useful tool to help with risk stratification, and will show right ventricular dysfunction in about half of all those patients with a normal BP.

Intervention

All patients with a PE should have IV access and oxygen. Unstable patients may also need intubation.

The vast majority of patients with a PE are clinically stable. Once diagnosed, get a full history that will enable you to assess the risks and benefits of anticoagulation. These patients should be monitored and admitted to the hospital. (Out-patient therapy for stable small PEs is being tried at some centers, but is not yet widespread.) You should start them on either heparin (80 mg/kg bolus followed by 18 u/kg/h) or LMWH (e.g. enoxaparin1 mg/kg) depending on your local standards.

Massive PE

Patients who present with shock or severe right heart dysfunction and who have no contraindications should be treated with thrombolytics (e.g. r-tPA 10 units IV over 2 minutes, repeat after 30 minutes). For patients in whom this fails, surgical options include either a transvenous catheter or surgical embolectomy, but the mortality in these groups is up to 50%.

Differential Diagnosis

Aortic dissection	Pneumonia
Costochondritis	Pneumothorax
MI	Rib fracture
Pericarditis	

Consultation

Talk with the PCP of all your patients with a PE. If the patient is unstable with a massive PE, the pulmonologist and ICU attending should be immediately consulted. In other centers, consult interventional radiology for a catheter embolectomy or CT surgery for a possible surgical embolectomy. Some of these options may not be available if you are working in a smaller hospital. In these cases you should discuss risks and benefits of transfer of the patient with your consultants, the patient and any family.

Disposition and Documentation

Stable patients should be admitted for anticoagulation and investigation into the etiology. Patients who are ill appearing or require thrombolytics should of course be admitted (if in the ED) or transferred (if on the floor) to the ICU. If you are considering thrombolysis, document your discussion with the patient and family.

Assessment of clinical risk of PE

Because a PE often presents with subtle clinical findings and a normal physical exam, the physician needs to use her index of suspicion to categorize the risk for the disease. This level of physician suspicion is

Table 12.3 Simplified Wells Score for Risk of PE	
Condition	Points
Previous PE or DVT	+1.5
Heart rate >100/min	+1.5
Recent surgery or immobilization	+1.5
Clinical signs of DVT	+3
Alternative diagnosis less likely than PE	+3
Hemoptysis	+1
Cancer	+1
Clinical Probability: 0–1 low 2–6 intermediate ≥7 high	

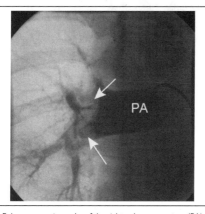

Figure 12.1 Pulmonary angiography of the right pulmonary artery (PA) demonstrating large filling defects (arrowed) in keeping with massive pulmonary emboli.

referred to as the pre-test risk. There have been attempts to combine the individual signs, symptoms, and tests into a scoring system, which classifies a risk of PE as small, medium, or high. On the basis of this score, the physician would decide whether or not to pursue a possible PE with a V/Q scan or CTA. A widely used prediction system is the Wells score (see Table 12.3). However, recent work has shown that a scoring system works about as well an empiric system. Because an empiric system is highly dependent on the physician's level of training, you should use an objective prediction rule (which is less influenced by a lack of experience) early on in your career.

Pulmonary Hypertension

Pulmonary hypertension is usually defined to be a mean pulmonary arterial pressure or more than 25 mmHg at rest or more than 30 mmHg with exercise. It is classified by the World Health Organization according to common pathobiological features (see box opposite). Primary pulmonary hypertension is the diagnosis in patients with pulmonary arterial hypertension of unexplained etiology. It is usually already established when the patient presents.

Presentation

- Breathlessness is the usual complaint although some patients present with exertional syncope (due to a fixed or reduced cardiac output) or angina (from right ventricular ischemia)
- Patients with pulmonary venous hypertension relating to left heart disease will often have symptoms of orthopnea and paroxysmal nocturnal dyspnea

Signs include:

- Elevated JVP with a large *a* wave (or a large *v* wave if severe tricuspid regurgitation)
- Low volume pulse
- Right ventricular heave (left parasternal)
- Loud pulmonary component of the second heart sound
- Systolic murmur (tricuspid regurgitation)
- Central and peripheral cyanosis
- Edema
- Ascites
- Signs of associated disease

Investigations

- *EKG:* Right ventricular hypertrophy is highly specific but has a low sensitivity. Right bundle branch block with anterior ST abnormalities can occur. Prominent P waves (P pulmonale) suggest right atrial enlargement

- *CXR:* This may show enlargement of the pulmonary artery and its major branches, and tapering of the peripheral arteries. The right atrium and ventricle are often enlarged
- *Bloods:* CBC, CMP, ESR, ABG, thrombophilia screen, autoimmune profile
- *Echocardiography:* Enlarged right ventricle with septal flattening. The ECHO should be able to give an estimate of the pulmonary artery systolic pressure

Further specialist investigations include:

- High resolution CT scan
- Lung perfusion scintigraphy
- Pulmonary function tests (particularly gas transfer)
- Hepatitis and HIV serology and viral titers
- Exercise testing
- Nocturnal oxygen saturation studies
- Cardiac catheterization and pulmonary angiography after specialist advice (increased risk).

Box 12.1 Classification and Causes

Pulmonary arterial hypertension
- Primary pulmonary hypertension (sporadic/familial)
- Associated with connective tissue disease, portal hypertension, HIV, drugs/toxins, other

Pulmonary venous hypertension
- Left-sided atrial or ventricular heart disease
- Left-sided valvular disease
- Extrinsic compression of central pulmonary veins

Pulmonary hypertension associated with respiratory disease/hypoxemia
- Chronic obstructive pulmonary disease
- Interstitial lung disease
- Sleep disordered breathing
- Alveolar hypoventilation disorders
- Chronic exposure to high altitude

Pulmonary hypertension due to chronic thrombotic/embolic disease
- Thromboembolic obstruction of proximal pulmonary arteries
- Obstruction of distal pulmonary arteries (PE, in situ thrombosis, sickle cell)

Pulmonary hypertension due to pulmonary vascular disorders
- Inflammatory (schistosomiasis, sarcoidosis, other)
- Pulmonary capillary hemangiomatosis.

Management

- Making the initial diagnosis of pulmonary hypertension is important but the actual cause may be difficult to identify quickly and is made after appropriate advice and investigation
- The management of patients presenting *de novo* with pulmonary hypertension includes appropriate use of oxygen to correct hypoxia, anticoagulation, and diuretic therapy
- Get specialist advice for patients known to have pulmonary hypertension who present unwell

The long-term management includes:

- Lifestyle changes (graded exercise activities)
- Anticoagulation with warfarin (INR 2.5)
- Diuretics (often high doses of loop diuretics are needed)
- Supplemental oxygen therapy

Box 12.2 Vasodilator Therapy in Primary Pulmonary Hypertension

During right heart cardiac catheterization, pulmonary hemodynamics are measured. Short-acting vasodilator therapy is used (inhaled nitric oxide, nebulized prostacyclin or intravenous adenosine). A positive response is defined as a >20% reduction in mean pulmonary artery pressure or pulmonary vascular resistance without a decrease in cardiac output. Patients who respond and who have a cardiac index >2.1 L/min/m^2, and/or mixed venous oxygen saturation >63% and/or right atrial pressure <10 mmHg should be considered for calcium channel blockers.

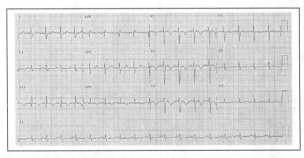

Figure 12.2 EKG in chronic severe pulmonary hypertension.
Right ventricular hypertrophy is demonstrated by right axis deviation, large R waves with T wave inversion in leads V1–3 and a prominent p wave (p pulmonale).

Other therapies will depend of the underlying cause.
They include:

- Vasodilator therapy (but less than 10% of patients benefit, see box)—high dose calcium channel blockers such as nifedipine (up to 240 mg/d) and diltiazem (up to 700 mg/d) are used
- Prostacyclins—continuous infusion of epoprostenol
- Endothelin receptor blockers—e.g. bosentan 125 mg bd
- Phosphodiesterase inhibitors—e.g. sildenafil, tadalafil
- Digoxin (to improve right ventricular function)
- Atrial septostomy
- Pulmonary thromboendarterectomy
- Heart-lung and lung transplantation.

Chapter 13

Systemic Emboli

Systemic Emboli

The embolization of thrombus or vegetation leads to signs and symptoms of obstruction of a coronary, cerebral, or peripheral artery.

Presentation

- Transient ischemic attack/stroke (common)
- Acute ischemia of a limb (painful, pulseless, pale, paralysis)
- MI or acute coronary syndrome
- Acute small bowel ischemia (superior mesenteric artery embolism)—abdominal pain, hypovolemia, few abdominal signs
- Acute renal failure (rare).

Investigations

This should be guided by the history and examination. Consider the following as a guide:

- CBC (anemia, platelet count/clumping), chemistry
- ESR and D-dimer
- Coagulation screen
- EKG (AF, MI)
- CXR (cardiomegaly)
- CT head if signs of a TIA or stroke (to exclude hemorrhage, intracranial mass)
- Carotid/peripheral artery Doppler ultrasound
- Doppler ultrasound of leg veins (DVT)
- Echocardiography (see p. 173).

Management

It is often necessary to manage the presenting condition before investigating the source of embolism (e.g. acute limb ischemia, small bowel ischemia). Patients should be anticoagulated if a cardiac source of embolism is demonstrated. However, the use of early anticoagulation in embolic stroke is controversial and should be initiated according to your own local hospital policy. Obtain a cardiothoracic consult if there is a PFO or ASD. In patients with a DVT who have contraindications to warfarin, get interventional radiology to place an inferior vena cava filter.

Box 13.1 Causes

- Carotid atheroma (common)
- Left atrial appendage thrombus
  - AF
  - Mitral stenosis
  - Impaired atrial function

Box 13.1 (Continued)

- Left ventricular thrombus (post infarct, cardiomyopathy, left ventricular aneurysm, non-compaction)
- Left heart valves
  - Prosthetic (endocarditis, thrombosis)
  - Native (aortic stenosis, mitral stenosis)
- Cardiac shunt with paradoxical embolism
  - Atrial septal defect (ASD)
  - Patent foramen ovale (PFO)
  - Ventricular septal defect (with raised right ventricular pressure)
- Aorta
  - Atheroma
  - Dissection (p. 144)
- Cardiac tumors (p. 240)
  - Myxoma
  - Other primary and secondary tumors (all are very rare).

Box 13.2 Echocardiography for Systemic Emboli

Indications for transthoracic echocardiography (TTE)

- Unexplained systemic embolism
- TTE is also indicated if clinical signs of endocarditis (p. 116), myxoma (p. 240)

In the absence of a cardiac history, EKG abnormalities or clinical signs, a TTE is unlikely to be useful.

Indications for transesophageal echocardiography (TEE)

- Non-diagnostic TTE
- Endocarditis suspected and not confirmed on TTE
- Suspected prosthetic valve dysfunction
- Suspected PFO or ASD

Paradoxical Emboli

These are systemic emboli which arise when emboli from the venous system cross an abnormal communication within the heart (usually via an ASD or PFO).

- A PFO is the most common cardiac abnormality found in young patients with unexplained stroke
- For a PFO to cause a systemic emboli the following triad is required:
  - The presence of a PFO

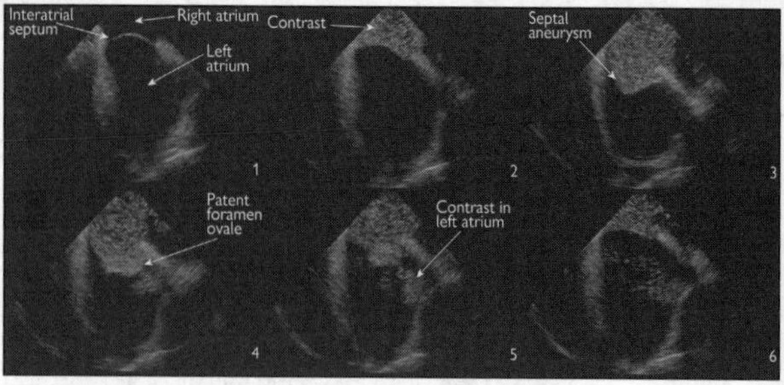

Figure 13.1 Intracardiac echocardiography study demonstrating passage of agitated saline contrast from the right atrium through a patent foramen ovale into the left atrium. The interatrial septum is aneurysmal.

- Raised right atrial pressure (permanent or transient, e.g. coughing, straining)
- Venous source of thrombosis (usually a deep vein thrombosis).

The diagnosis is best made with echocardiography, sometimes using saline contrast.

- Assesses right to left shunting using the Valsalva maneuver to increase right atrial pressure. In a normal study no bubbles should cross to the left heart
- If the TTE is positive, a TEE is still needed to assess the atrial septum for suitability of device closure
- False negatives may occur: on TTE due to poor image quality; with TEE due to poor Valsalva maneuver and failure to increase right atrial pressure
- Injecting saline contrast via the femoral vein increases the diagnostic accuracy (blood is directed via the eustachian valve towards the PFO).

Chapter 14

Cardiac Issues in Pregnancy

Introduction

For patients with known cardiac disease, pregnancy should ideally be planned and undertaken following consideration of risks to the mother and fetus. In some cases it may be necessary to alter or stop treatment prior to conception (e.g. warfarin and ACE inhibitors).

Pregnancy may also be associated with new presentations of heart disease. Remember that pregnancy can:

- Unmask pre-existing conditions
- Exacerbate pre-existing conditions
- Precipitate new conditions.

Although death during pregnancy is very rare (approximately 1 per 50,000 pregnancies) cardiac disease is the most common cause (e.g. cardiomyopathy, aortic dissection, myocardial infarction, complications of pulmonary hypertension).

Normal Physiological Changes in Pregnancy

One of the challenges to diagnosing pregnancy-related heart disease is to distinguish pathological features from adaptive changes in cardiovascular function. Circulating volume, heart rate, stroke volume, and consequently cardiac output increase markedly in the first 16 weeks, plateau and then increase further in the weeks before term. The following are all consistent with normal pregnancy:

- Fatigue
- Shortness of breath
- Palpitation, re-entrant SVT
- Atrial and ventricular premature beats
- Raised jugular venous pressure
- Pedal edema
- Sinus tachycardia (~100 bpm)
- Full volume, collapsing pulse
- 3rd heart sound
- Systolic flow murmur.

Clinical Indicators of Pathological States

- Chest pain
- Severe dyspnea
- Orthopnea, paroxysmal nocturnal dyspnea
- Sinus tachycardia >100 at rest
- AF/atrial flutter
- Ventricular tachycardia
- Hypotension
- Pulmonary edema
- Pleural effusion

Avoid drugs if possible, and use the fewest drugs in the smallest dose, *but* do not deny appropriate management because of pregnancy. Remember, if the mother is compromised, so is the fetus. Obtain EARLY advice from an obstetrician with expertise in managing high risk pregnancies, as well as a cardiologist.

Heart Failure in Pregnancy

Heart failure accounts for 25% of all cardiac deaths in pregnancy. Mortality is up to 10% when the left ventricular ejection fraction is ≤20%. Because of this very high mortality, consider termination if heart failure occurs early in pregnancy.

Causes

- Dilated cardiomyopathy
- Underlying structural conditions, e.g. valvular disease
- Peripartum cardiomyopathy is clinically indistinguishable from other dilated cardiomyopathies but by definition occurs only in the last month of pregnancy or up to 6 months post partum, *in the absence of any other cardiac pathology*. LV dysfunction persists in 50% of patients and there is a significant risk of recurrence in subsequent pregnancies even when the LV function has initially returned to normal. If LV function does not return to normal, the risk of death in any subsequent pregnancy is about 20%.

Acute Management

The management is similar to other forms of heart failure, namely bed rest and diuretics (see p. 63). The vasodilator hydralazine is often used. Because of the risk of renal agenesis, ACE inhibitors should be avoided until after delivery.

Aortic Disease in Pregnancy

The major concern is aortic dissection, which is usually associated with underlying aortic disease.

Causes and Associations

- Marfan syndrome, especially with aortic root >4 cm (p. 149)
- Turner's syndrome (assisted conception) or mosaic Turner's ~2% risk of dissection in pregnancy

- Aortic coarctation (whether corrected or not)
- Bicuspid aortic valve with dilated aortic root. However, the risk of dissection in pregnancy is only slightly higher than in the general population.

General Management

Patients at risk should have pre-conception evaluation of the aorta with echocardiography and/or magnetic resonance. During pregnancy, further monitoring is warranted. Beta-blockers are advised to reduce the risk of root dilation. If there is evidence of aortic dilatation, a caesarian section should be undertaken to minimize hemodynamic stresses.

Acute Aortic Dissection in Pregnancy

See pp. 146–148 for general management. Use a pelvic wedge when the patient is supine to prevent IVC obstruction. The blood pressure should be controlled with beta-blockers and hydralazine. (Sodium nitroprusside risks fetal toxicity and should *not* be used.) Consult with the obstetricians regarding the timing of the caesarian section.

Acute MI in Pregnancy

Acute MI in pregnancy is rare, occurring in 1 per 10,000 pregnancies. This incidence is increasing, probably may be due to the rising maternal age. Mortality is high (37–50%), particularly if the infarct occurs late in pregnancy. The diagnosis is made using conventional criteria (p. 43). Troponin I is not affected by normal pregnancy and is the marker of choice for myocardial necrosis in pregnancy.

Acute Management

There are few data to guide treatment. The risk from MI needs to be weighed against the risks of treatment (to both mother and fetus). Give all patients aspirin and beta-blockers. The treatment of choice is PCI in an ST elevation MI, and the consequence of not treating carries a high risk of both maternal and fetal death. Although there are little data on the use of newer antiplatelet agents in pregnancy, there are reports of successful completion of pregnancy following primary angioplasty.

Systemic thrombolysis should not be given late in pregnancy because of the risk of premature labor and potentially catastrophic bleeding. However, in the presence of a large anterolateral acute MI, thrombolysis should be considered if primary angioplasty is not available, since the consequence of not treating carries such a high risk of maternal and fetal demise.

Pulmonary Embolism in Pregnancy

Venous thromboembolism is the second most common cause of maternal death, and poor management is implicated in many. Appropriate investigations should not be withheld because of pregnancy. Patients should be anticoagulated pending a confirmed diagnosis. CT scans of the chest and perfusion scans carry a low risk to the fetus and should not be withheld.

Acute Management

Low molecular weight heparin can be used but altered pharmacokinetics in pregnancy mean that doses may need to be altered according to levels of anti-Xa (0.6–1.0 units/mL). For life-threatening massive PE, obtain an emergent consultation with interventional radiology or a cardiothoracic surgeon. Options include intra-pulmonary thrombolysis, catheter (percutaneous) disruption of embolus, or surgical thrombectomy. Where embolic episodes continue despite therapeutic anti-coagulation, consider a temporary caval filter.

Valvular Heart Disease in Pregnancy

Mitral Stenosis

Increased heart rate (decreased diastolic filling time) and increased circulating volume both serve to increase left atrial pressure and may precipitate acute pulmonary edema. New or rapid AF will have similar effects.

Treatment

- Diuretics (avoid excessive diuresis because of the risk of hypovolemia)
- Beta-blockers for rate control
- Anticoagulate with heparin (if in AF and/or left atrial dilatation)
- Percutaneous (balloon) mitral valvuloplasty for severe mitral stenosis that is refractory to medical treatment.

Aortic Stenosis

This is usually due to a bicuspid aortic valve. The increased cardiac output required early in pregnancy can lead to problems due to the fixed LV outflow. Symptoms include SOB, syncope, and chest pain. When these occur with severe aortic stenosis, consider delivery or palliative balloon valvuloplasty.

Valvular Regurgitation

Mitral and aortic regurgitation are generally well tolerated during pregnancy, and the decreased afterload is often beneficial in reducing the degree of regurgitation. When symptoms do occur, diuretics are the mainstay of treatment. ACE inhibitors should be avoided.

Arrhythmias in Pregnancy

Hormonal and hemodynamic changes may predispose pregnant women to arrhythmias. These changes may also cause paroxysmal tachycardias to become symptomatic when they otherwise would go unnoticed by the patient. Remember that DC cardioversion is safe in pregnancy.

Re-entry Tachycardias

- Treat as for non-pregnant (p. 95)
- Vagal maneuvers
- Adenosine, verapamil, flecainide have been used successfully
- When there is hemodynamic compromise, proceed to DC cardioversion (p. 256)

AF and Atrial Flutter

- Underlying cardiac disease likely and should be investigated
- Cardiovert if compromised and <24 hour duration
- Anticoagulate with low molecular-weight heparin
- Give beta-blockers to control rate
- Involve cardiologist and high risk obstetrician in management decisions.

Ventricular Tachycardia

- This requires DC cardioversion acutely
- Once stable, keep on telemetry and further evaluate the cause. Subsequent management will depend on the underlying disease
- Involve both the cardiologist and high risk obstetrician.

Hypertension in Pregnancy

There are three types of hypertension in pregnancy, which is usually defined as a BP >140 systolic or 90 mmHg diastolic:

- Chronic hypertension
- Gestational hypertension
- Pre-eclampsia.

Control of chronic hypertension (i.e., hypertension which was diagnosed prior to or in early pregnancy) may deteriorate and require alteration to treatment. For example, ACE inhibitors are contraindicated in pregnancy and should be discontinued prior to conception.

Gestational hypertension occurs late in pregnancy (last trimester). Pre-eclampsia tends to occur in younger women with onset after 20 weeks' gestation. Consider this in any case of an abrupt onset of edema and proteinuria or hypertension. A raised plasma uric acid will distinguish pre-eclampsia from chronic hypertension. Resolution following delivery is the rule.

The drugs most commonly used to control hypertension in pregnancy are methyldopa (250 mg TDS po initially) and/or hydralazine (5–10 mg IV, repeated after 30 minutes in severe hypertension) with calcium antagonists and beta-blockers as second line agents.

Magnesium sulfate is given in pre-eclampsia to prevent seizures. Avoid nitroprusside because of fetal toxicity.

Anticoagulation in Pregnancy

Sub-specialist advice should be sought and decisions made after consideration of case-specific issues.

Anticoagulation in pregnancy, particularly for prosthetic valves presents a difficult problem, with few data available for guidance. Warfarin carries the high risks of teratogenicity (first trimester), fetal hemorrhage (especially in third trimester) and fetal loss throughout pregnancy. Heparin use has been implicated in prosthetic valve thrombosis. LMW heparin is preferred to unfractionated heparin, because anti-Xa levels can be monitored. It should be given as a bd regime.

The three main therapeutic options are:
1. Heparin/LMW heparin plus aspirin throughout pregnancy.
2. Warfarin throughout pregnancy, changing to heparin at 38 weeks.
3. Heparin/LMW heparin plus aspirin in 1st trimester, changing to warfarin until 38 weeks when heparin is recommenced.

> ### Box 14.2 DC Cardioversion in Pregnancy
> - Place a wedge under the right hip to avoid IVC compression*
> - Use lowest energy shock
> - Direct the paddles away from fetus
> - No reports of iatrogenic fetal VF
> - … but, check fetal heart rate post-cardioversion
>
> * Procedures or investigations that usually require the patient to be supine should be done in a lateral position or with the aid of a wedge to support the pelvis and avoid IVC compression by the gravid uterus, with consequent syncope.

Chapter 15

Adult Congenital Heart Disease

Introduction

Congenital heart defects are the most common type of birth defect, affecting 8 of every 1,000 newborns. Most of these defects are simple conditions that are easily fixed or need no treatment.

A small number of babies are more complex and may require intervention soon after birth. Most children with complex heart defects grow to adulthood and can live active, productive lives because their heart defects have been effectively treated.

Today in the United States, about 1 million adults are living with congenital heart defects. They may need to pay special attention to certain issues that their condition could affect such as pregnancy, and preventing infection during routine health procedures. Common presentations in emergency situations include:

- Arrhythmia
- Heart failure
- Endocarditis

—all with high mortality. Special expertise is needed for optimal management.

Atrial Septal Defect (ASD)

An ASD is a direct communication between the two atria that permits blood flow to the chamber under lower pressure (usually from left to right atrium). Shunting of blood flow back into the venous circulation eventually results in enlargement of the right atrium and ventricle and increased pulmonary blood flow. The most common defect is an ostium scundum defect; the second most common is an ostium premum defect.

The Unoperated Patient

Clinical features result from:

- Increased pulmonary blood flow
- Inability to increase cardiac output adequately because of the systemic-to-pulmonary shunting
- Paradoxical thromboembolism
- AF or flutter, related to atrial dilatation.

Presentation

- Many are asymptomatic
- Symptomatic adults usually present with SOB or palpitation age 20–40
- May present as an emergency with stroke, heart failure, or AF with rapid ventricular response.

Signs

- Fixed splitting of the 2nd heart sound
- Pulmonary ejection murmur (due to increased flow)
- Cyanosis (uncommon; occurs in large defects with pulmonary hypertension).

Investigations

CXR: Cardiomegaly, right atrial dilatation and prominent pulmonary arteries are common with large shunts.

EKG: Right axis deviation and incomplete RBBB are typical findings in patients with significant defects.

There is often an atrial arrhythmia (AF, flutter).

Management

- Acute management of stroke, heart failure, or AF as in the non-ACHD setting
- An ASD that gives rise to right ventricular enlargement should be closed either surgically or with a percutaneous technique. This does not need to be done urgently
- If there is a large defect, with established pulmonary hypertension, cyanosis and Eisenmenger syndrome, closure may be too hazardous.

The Operated Patient

After ASD closure, patients are usually symptom-free. However, they can present with atrial arrhythmias and heart failure especially when the defect has been closed late in life and the pulmonary artery pressure has been elevated prior to surgery. Complete heart block or sinus node dysfunction can also occur after closure.

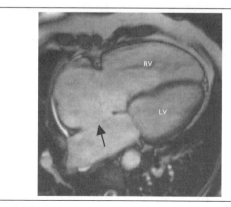

Figure 15.1 Cardiac magnetic resonance image of an atrial septal defect. Note the partial absence of atrial septum (arrowed) and the dilated RV.

Ventricular Septal Defect (VSD)

A VSD permits blood flow between the ventricles (usually from left to right) leading to an increase in pulmonary blood flow and enlargement of the left atrium and ventricle. The size of the VSD and the pulmonary vascular resistance determine the degree and direction of the shunt.

The Unoperated Patient—Problems

- Pulmonary hypertension can result from a large defect with significant left-to-right shunt and may become permanent due to chronic pulmonary vascular changes
- Cyanosis occurs when increased pulmonary vascular resistance eventually leads to a right-to-left shunt (Eisenmenger syndrome, p. 200)
- Heart failure from left ventricular dysfunction due to long-term volume overload
- Atrial and ventricular arrhythmias due to chamber enlargement and stretch
- Aortic regurgitation (p. 135), even with small VSDs, due to the potential proximity of the defect to the aortic valve
- Increased risk of endocarditis (p. 116)—all patients with VSDs
- Pregnancy is usually well tolerated in patients with a small or moderate VSD but carries a high risk in patients with pulmonary vascular disease (Eisenmenger syndrome, p. 200).

Acute presentation

Patients may present acutely with endocarditis, atrial and ventricular arrhythmias, or heart failure.

Signs

- Coarse pansystolic heart murmur at left sternal border ('the louder the VSD murmur, the smaller the defect')
- Left ± right ventricular heave
- Cyanosis if Eisenmenger syndrome has developed (p. 200).

Investigations

CXR:
Small defect: usually normal
Moderate defect: cardiomegaly, increased pulmonary marking
Large defect (with Eisenmenger syndrome): oligemic lung fields, enlarged proximal pulmonary arteries
EKG: Broad P wave, signs of LV enlargement or RV hypertrophy (Eisenmenger syndrome), arrhythmia.

Management

- Acute presenting problems managed as in the non-ACHD setting

- Nearly all VSDs should be closed to alleviate LV enlargement, prevent the development of irreversible pulmonary artery disease and to reduce the risk of aortic regurgitation and bacterial endocarditis (one exception is small uncomplicated VSDs).

The Operated Patient

- Usually symptom-free but can present with atrial or ventricular arrhythmia or heart failure, especially when the defect has been closed late in life and the pulmonary artery pressure has been elevated
- Complete heart block can occur after closure
- Pulmonary vascular disease can progress, regress, or remain stable post-operatively.

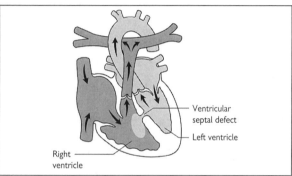

Right ventricle

Ventricular septal defect

Left ventricle

Figure 15.2 Diagram of a ventricular septal defect.

Box 15.1 Restrictive and Non-restrictive VSD

Restrictive VSDs 'restrict' the flow across the defect. They are thus small VSDs ($<1/_3$ of the aortic root diameter), and there is a pressure gradient between the left and right ventricles. RV pressures and pulmonary resistance are normal.

Moderately restrictive VSDs are about ½ the size of the aortic valve, with moderate to severe shunting early in the disease process. RV pressures are increased, but not to systemic levels. Pulmonary resistance can be raised, and the left atrium and ventricle can be dilated due to volume overload.

Non-restrictive VSDs are large, resulting in equal left and right ventricular pressures. The pulmonary circulation is subject to systemic pressures and significantly increased flow, which leads to increased pulmonary resistance within the first years of life. This reduces the left-to-right shunt and continued pulmonary vascular changes ultimately result in reversal of the shunt (right-to-left) and Eisenmenger syndrome (p. 200).

Atrioventricular Septal Defect (AVSD)

The term AVSD covers a spectrum of anomalies at the junction between the atria and ventricles:

- The defect can consist only of an ASD (ostium primum) or can include an inlet-type VSD, which can be restrictive or non-restrictive
- Additionally, the atrioventricular valves (mitral and tricuspid) are often abnormal and can be regurgitant
- AVSDs occur in 35% of patients with Down syndrome.

Physiological Consequences

- Generally similar to the condition of an isolated ASD or VSD and relate to the degree of left-to-right shunting and the presence or absence of pulmonary hypertension
- The abnormality of the AV valves can result in additional problems, including heart failure and atrial arrhythmia.

Repair

Following AVSD repair, mitral or tricuspid regurgitation, or stenosis, subaortic stenosis and complete AV block can occur.

Patent Ductus Arteriosus (PDA)

A PDA represents a persistent communication between the descending aorta and the proximal left pulmonary artery.

- There is a left-to-right shunt with increased pulmonary flow leading to enlargement of the left atrium and ventricle
- Small ducts cause a murmur without hemodynamic effects
- Large ducts lead to pulmonary hypertension and pulmonary vascular disease, ultimately resulting in Eisenmenger syndrome and a right-to-left shunt across the PDA into the *descending* aorta. This results in differential cyanosis (reduced lower body oxygen saturations with maintained upper body saturation).

Signs

Continuous (systolic and diastolic) murmur at upper left sternal border; long ejection systolic murmur with small PDAs.

Acute Presentation

Rare—endarteritis (like endocarditis) is the main cause.

Management

- Endarteritis managed as for endocarditis in the non-ACHD setting (p. 117)
- Closure of PDA is indicated if left heart enlarged or when a murmur is present (to reduce the small risk of endarteritis).

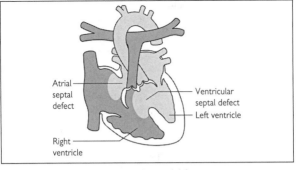

Figure 15.3 Diagram of an atrioventricular septal defect.

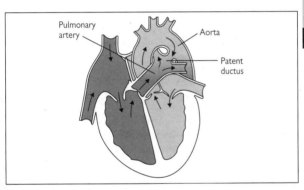

Figure 15.4 Diagram of a patent ductus arteriosus.

Aortic Coarctation

Aortic coarctation is a narrowing of the aorta in the region of the ligamentum arteriosum, just distal to the left subclavian artery. If severe, the lower body relies on collateral vessels via the intercostal arteries for perfusion. Complete occlusion is also possible. A 'simple' coarctation is one without other cardiac lesions. A 'complex' coarctation is associated with other defects such as a VSD or left sided obstructive lesion (e.g. aortic stenosis). At least 50% of patients with coarctation have a bicuspid aortic valve.

The Unoperated Patient

Risks

- Upper body hypertension
- Heart failure from long-standing LV pressure load
- Aortic rupture or dissection
- Infective endocarditis
- Stroke from an associated ruptured berry aneurysm + hypertension
- Premature coronary artery disease.

Signs

- Upper limb hypertension and differential arm-leg pulses. Blood pressure measurement in the right arm and a leg is necessary in all new patients with hypertension. A pressure difference of ≥20 mmHg may suggest coarctation
- Continuous murmur in the interscapular region.

Investigations

EKG: Left ventricular hypertrophy.

CXR: Look for narrowing of the aorta at the site of coarctation with dilatation of the vessel before and after the coarctation, and rib notching caused by erosions of the inferior edge of the ribs by enlarged intercostal arteries.

CT: This provides good visualization of location and severity using contrast and reconstructed images.

MRI: Excellent visualization of anatomy, possible aneurysm formation and, using contrast angiography, 3D visualization of the geometry and collaterals. Velocity measurements can assess the degree of stenosis.

Management

- Acute consequences managed as in the non-ACHD setting
- Surgical repair or stenting of the stenosis may be indicated if significant gradient across coarctation (>20 mmHg) ± proximal hypertension.

The Operated Patient

- Re-coarctation and aneurysm formation (often intercostal) at the site of repair are not uncommon; aneurysm rupture presents acutely
- Other aortic wall complications are frequent
- Hypertension can persist or develop in adulthood and needs to be treated aggressively because of the risk of atherosclerosis
- The need for endocarditis prophylaxis remains.

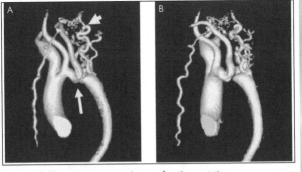

Figure 15.5 Magnetic resonance angiogram of aortic coarctation.
(A) AP view showing site of coarctation (long arrow), enlarged head and neck vessels and extensive collateral circulation to the descending aorta (short arrow).
(B) rotated view showing complete nature of coarctation.

Transposition of the Great Arteries (TGA)

- The aorta arises from the RV and the pulmonary artery from the LV
- TGA can be associated with other lesions, e.g. VSD or coarctation
- TGA is incompatible with life without treatment in the first few days.

Atrial Switch Operation

- The most common operation among adults with TGA is an 'atrial switch operation' (either Mustard or Senning operation, p. 206)
- The atrial blood flow has been 'switched' in a way that the RV receives the pulmonary venous blood and the LV receives the systemic venous blood; however, the RV remains the systemic ventricle.

Arterial Switch Operation (p. 204)

The atrial switch operation has been replaced by the 'arterial switch operation' in which the aorta and pulmonary artery are switched to the anatomically correct position, with the LV connected to the aorta and the RV to the pulmonary artery (the LV becomes the systemic ventricle).

The Patient After Atrial Switch Operation

- There is a significant morbidity from arrhythmia related to extensive atrial surgery: especially common are bradyarrhythmias (due to sinus node dysfunction resulting in a slow junctional escape rhythm) and tachyarrhythmias (atrial flutter)

- RV dysfunction is common, since the right ventricle is not built to support the systemic circulation
- Tricuspid regurgitation can accompany right heart failure
- Obstruction of the atrial pathways ('baffle obstruction') can lead to systemic or pulmonary venous congestion.

Signs

- Systolic heart murmur from tricuspid regurgitation
- Heart failure
- Peripheral edema and ascites from systemic venous congestion.

Investigations

- *EKG*—Right axis deviation, RV hypertrophy, atrial arrhythmias
- *CXR*—Cardiomegaly, pulmonary congestion.

Management

- The complexity of arrhythmia management, including pacing, and the difficulty in assessing RV function requires a specialist referral center
- Thorough assessment of RV and tricuspid valve function, heart rhythm, and the function of the intra-atrial venous pathways is paramount
- Therapeutic options include catheterization techniques (balloon dilatation and stenting for pathway obstructions) and surgical procedures (tricuspid valve repair/replacement or even conversion to the arterial switch operation, for selected patients)
- The end of the therapeutic spectrum is heart transplantation.

If pacing is required for bradycardia, this must be performed by those with prior experience of the procedure in this class of patients, since placement of the leads within the atria and into the left (pulmonary) ventricle can be immensely difficult.

The Patient After Arterial Switch Operation

- Arrhythmias are less common and ventricular function is usually well preserved
- Suture lines in the pulmonary trunk can cause stenosis
- Peripheral pulmonary artery stenosis can be caused by the position of the pulmonary bifurcation anterior to the ascending aorta
- Progressive dilatation of the aortic root (former pulmonary root) can cause aortic regurgitation
- Coronary artery reimplantation may result in ostial coronary stenosis and ischemia.

Signs

- Ejection systolic heart murmur from pulmonary artery stenosis
- Diastolic heart murmur from aortic regurgitation.

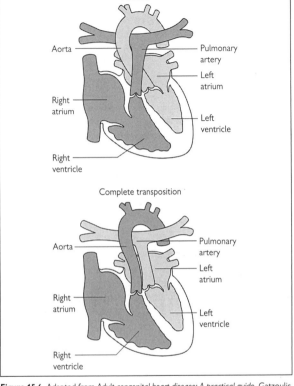

Figure 15.6 Adapted from *Adult congenital heart disease: A practical guide*. Gatzoulis MA, et al. (eds). © 2005 Wiley-Blackwell.

Investigations

EKG—Signs of myocardial ischemia and RV hypertrophy.

Management

The main issue in the care of patients after arterial switch operation is to exclude significant pulmonary artery stenosis, myocardial ischemia, and aortic valve regurgitation. All these situations warrant intervention.

Congenitally Corrected Transposition of the Great Arteries (ccTGA)

In ccTGA the ventricles are 'inverted.' Systemic venous return enters the left ventricle which then ejects into the pulmonary artery.

Pulmonary venous return enters the right ventricle which fills the aorta. The circulation is therefore physiologically corrected but the right ventricle is supporting the systemic circulation.

ccTGA is often associated with other defects, e.g. systemic (tricuspid) atrioventricular valve abnormalities and regurgitation, VSD, subpulmonary stenosis, and complete heart block. ccTGA can occur with dextrocardia.

The Unoperated Patient

- Progressive RV dysfunction is common as it is not designed to support the systemic circulation
- Risk of bradyarrhythmias (complete AV block) and tachyarrhythmias (atrial arrhythmia pp. 82–86 or SVT secondary to WPW syndrome, p. 96)
- Patients with a VSD and pulmonary stenosis can be cyanotic.

The Operated Patient

Patients may have been operated for their associated lesions. Common procedures are:
- VSD closure
- Implantation of a conduit from the LV to the pulmonary artery
- Systemic (tricuspid) atrioventricular valve replacement.

A corrective procedure would be the 'double switch operation' (combination of an atrial and arterial switch operation). As for atrial switch operations, atrial arrhythmias are common following this.

Signs

Listen for a systolic heart murmur. This may a VSD, pulmonary stenosis, or tricuspid regurgitation; the specific lesion is difficult to differentiate clinically.

Investigations

- EKG—Arrhythmia (complete AV block, atrial arrhythmia)
- CXR—Dextrocardia (20% of patients), cardiomegaly.

Management

- Preservation of systemic (right) ventricular function is crucial
- Tricuspid regurgitation has to be treated surgically (valve replacement) before ventricular dysfunction becomes irreversible
- Symptomatic bradycardia or chronotropic incompetence is an indication for pacemaker implantation
- Atrial arrhythmias are common after atrial surgery or with severe tricuspid regurgitation. They are not well tolerated in the setting of a systemic RV, especially with dysfunction and tricuspid regurgitation
- Endocarditis prophylaxis is necessary in all patients.

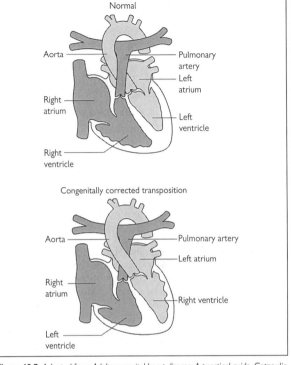

Figure 15.7 Adapted from *Adult congenital heart disease: A practical guide*. Gatzoulis MA, et al. (eds). © 2005 Wiley-Blackwell.

Tetralogy of Fallot (ToF)

Tetralogy of Fallot consists of:
- A large VSD
- Right ventricular outflow tract obstruction (RVOTO)
- Right ventricular hypertrophy
- An overriding aorta.

The physiological consequences are determined by the degree of RVOTO which in turn determines the magnitude of pulmonary blood flow. Significant RVOTO leads to a right-to-left shunt and cyanosis. Survival to adulthood in unoperated patients with ToF is rare.

The Operated or Repaired Patient

- Surgical repair includes VSD closure and relief of the RVOTO and may involve patching of the pulmonary valve annulus, which can lead to pulmonary regurgitation
- Pulmonary regurgitation in turn may lead to right ventricular enlargement and dysfunction and is associated with VT and sudden death. However, the majority of patients tolerate the regurgitation well
- Atrial arrhythmias are not uncommon especially if right atrial enlargement is present.

Signs
There is a diastolic murmur (from pulmonary or aortic regurgitation) and a systolic murmur (from residual RVOTO or VSD).

Investigations
- *EKG*—complete RBBB, QRS prolongation
- *CXR*—cardiomegaly.

Management

- Pulmonary valve replacement should be considered for patients with severe pulmonary regurgitation and right ventricular dilatation. New percutaneous techniques, using stent-mounted pericardial valves, show promise in selected patients.
- The development of arrhythmias (VT and atrial flutter/fibrillation) warrants both full electrophysiologic assessment and a thorough review of the hemodynamics.

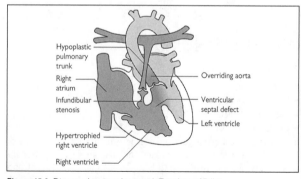

Figure 15.8 Diagram showing a heart with Tetralogy of Fallot.
Adapted from *Adult congenital heart disease: A practical guide.* Gatzoulis MA, et al. (eds). © 2005 Wiley-Blackwell.

The Single Ventricle

Hearts with an anatomically or functionally single ventricle receive the systemic and pulmonary venous blood in 'one' ventricle, which can be of predominantly left or right ventricular morphology. The ventricle pumps blood into the pulmonary artery (when not atretic) and the aorta.

The best situation is when blood flows unrestricted into a well-functioning ventricle, which pumps an equivalent amount of blood into the lungs and systemic circulation. In this situation, excessive pulmonary blood flow is avoided by an obstruction of the pulmonary outflow tract. If pulmonary outflow tract obstruction is not present, excessive blood flow into the lungs will lead to pulmonary hypertension and the Eisenmenger syndrome (p. 200).

Severe pulmonary outflow tract obstruction with reduced pulmonary blood flow causes cyanosis (p. 199).

Surgery in patients with single ventricles is always palliative and aims to secure adequate pulmonary and systemic blood flow and maintain systemic ventricular function.

Surgery for Single Ventricles

- Aorto-pulmonary shunts are commonly performed in early infancy to improve pulmonary blood flow. As the single ventricle continues to pump blood into both the aorta and pulmonary arteries, volume overload remains a problem
- Pulmonary artery banding is performed when pulmonary blood flow is unobstructed, to protect against pulmonary hypertension
- Systemic venous to pulmonary artery connections like the Glenn shunt (p. 205) or the Fontan operation (p. 205) are performed as definitive palliations to improve pulmonary blood flow and separate the pulmonary from the systemic circulation while unloading the systemic ventricle.

The Patient After Fontan Operation

Many adult patients with a single ventricle have undergone Fontan operations (p. 205). Following this operation, all systemic venous return is diverted to the pulmonary circulation without employing a subpulmonary ventricle. Blood flow to the lungs, therefore, is only driven by systemic venous pressure. Fontan patients are at risk of various complications related to surgery and/or the abnormal circulatory physiology persisting after surgery.

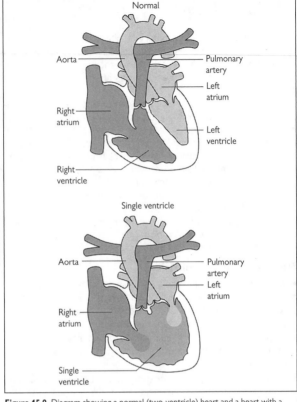

Figure 15.9 Diagram showing a normal (two-ventricle) heart and a heart with a single ventricle.
Adapted from *Adult congenital heart disease: A practical guide.* Gatzoulis MA, et al. (eds). © 2005 Wiley-Blackwell.

Complications After Fontan Operation

Arrhythmias

- Sinus node dysfunction may warrant pacemaker implantation.
- Atrial flutter/fibrillation related to scarring from surgery, or to atrial distension from high venous pressure.
- Atrial arrhythmias in Fontan patients need prompt treatment as they can cause profound hemodynamic deterioration.

Thromboembolism

This is associated with sluggish venous blood flow.

Protein losing enteropathy (PLE)

Occurs in 10% of Fontan patients and is characterized by intestinal protein loss leading to low serum protein levels and subsequently to peripheral edema and ascites.

Deterioration of ventricular function

This is the often the natural history of this anomaly, especially if the ventricle is of RV morphology.

Hepatic dysfunction

Resulting from high hepatic venous pressure.

Cyanosis

From persistent right-to-left shunting.

Signs

- A 'good' Fontan patient has no murmurs and a single 2nd heart sound (systolic murmurs can indicate atrioventricular valve incompetence)
- Peripheral edema (from heart failure or PLE).

Investigations

EKG—arrhythmia
CXR—cardiomegaly, atrial enlargement
Bloods—abnormal LFT, low protein/albumin suggestive of PLE.

Management

- Fontan patients are one of the most challenging group of patients in cardiology and require close follow up by tertiary center specialists
- Treatment aims to maintain optimal pulmonary and systemic circulation and to preserve ventricular function.

The Cyanosed Patient

Cyanosis is common in adults with congenital heart disease due to right-to-left shunting or decreased pulmonary blood flow. The resulting hypoxemia leads to adaptive mechanisms to increase oxygen delivery to the tissues. These include a rightward shift in the oxy-hemoglobin binding curve and an increased hemoglobin concentration (secondary erythrocytosis, not polycythemia).

Symptoms related to hypoxia include dyspnea at rest or on exertion and chest pain. Other symptoms result from the multi-organ consequences.

The Multi-organ Consequences of Cyanosis

Hematological

- Erythrocytosis
- Iron deficiency (high demand, dietary, or induced by inappropriate venesections)

- Coagulopathy, bleeding diathesis, thrombocytopenia, impaired clotting function.

Neurological

- Brain injury from paradoxical embolism, hemorrhage, abscesses.

Renal

- Hypoxemia-induced glomerulopathy (look for hematuria and proteinuria)
- Nephrolithiasis (uric acid).

Rheumatological

- Gout
- Osteoarthropathy.

Management

Venesections should be considered in cyanosed patients only if:

- There are severe symptoms of hyperviscosity syndrome (e.g. headache, dizziness, fatigue, visual disturbances, tinnitus and myalgia) despite correcting any dehydration, and the hematocrit is greater than 65%
- Surgery is planned and hematocrit is greater than 65%.

Venesection procedure

- 250–500 mL of blood should be removed over 45 minutes
- Volume replacement with 5% dextrose
- Use IV 'air filters' (to reduce the risk of systemic air embolus)
- Blood pressure and heart rate monitoring are required.

Iron deficiency

These patients require oral or IV iron supplements.

Anticoagulation

There is no general consensus on routine anticoagulation, and a multidisciplinary approach is best.

Eisenmenger Syndrome

Eisenmenger syndrome is a pathophysiological condition resulting from adult congenital heart disease. Uncorrected left-to-right shunting and progressive pulmonary hypertension eventually leads to a reversal of the shunt and cyanosis when the right-sided pressure exceeds the systemic pressure. VSD, AVSD, and large PDAs are responsible for 80% of cases. Eisenmenger patients exhibit signs and symptoms related to chronic cyanosis (p. 199) and are at risk of complications related to pulmonary hypertension (p. 166).

Signs

Look for cyanosis and listen for a loud second heart sound.

Investigations

- *EKG*—right ventricular hypertrophy
- *CXR*—oligemic lung fields, enlarged proximal pulmonary arteries.

Acute Presentation

- Progressive heart failure
- Atrial arrhythmias
- Angina
- Syncope and sudden cardiac death
- Hemoptysis and intrapulmonary bleeding
- Pulmonary artery thrombosis (embolism or *in situ* thrombosis).

Management

Hemoptysis/intrapulmonary bleeding

- Bed rest
- CXR and CT scan to determine extent of hemorrhage
- FBC (repeatedly if continuous bleeding is suspected)
- Monitoring of oxygen saturation, blood pressure, diuresis
- Embolization of culprit vessels identified by angiography.

Anticoagulation

- To prevent recurrent embolic events
- No general consensus on routine anticoagulation (bleeding diathesis).

Treatment of pulmonary hypertension

While pulmonary vasodilator therapy with agents such as prostacyclin analogues and endothelin antagonists are established forms of therapy in *primary* pulmonary hypertension, placebo controlled trials on the efficacy and safety of these drugs in Eisenmenger patients are under way. Early observational studies are encouraging.

Box 15.2 Rules in the Care of Eisenmenger Patients

- Avoid *hypovolemia* and *dehydration*
- Avoid *non-cardiac surgery* and general *anesthesia* if possible
- General anesthesia always needs to be performed by an experienced anesthesiologist
- Post-operative care should be managed in the ICU
- Use IV air filters or a bubble trap for any intravenous line

Arrhythmias

Arrhythmias are very common in adults with congenital heart disease as part of the natural history or resulting from surgery and or progressive residual hemodynamic lesions. Arrhythmias in these patients are associated with significant morbidity and mortality. Both the detection and treatment of arrhythmia in adults with congenital heart disease can be challenging.

Atypical Atrial Flutter and Intra-atrial Re-entry Tachycardia (IART)

IART is usually caused by atrial stretch or previous extensive atrial surgery (such as a Fontan, Mustard, or Senning procedure). Intra-atrial excitation circuits around electrical barriers such as scars and suture lines cause rapid atrial heart rate or flutter. Atrioventricular conduction may be normal in relatively young adults, allowing for a fast 1:1 conduction and a fast ventricular rate leading to hemodynamic compromise.

Treatment

Radiofrequency ablation can block the circuits and potentially treat the arrhythmia. Electrophysiologists with special expertise in CHD are required for these demanding procedures.

Ventricular Tachycardia (VT)

VT is commonly associated with previous ventricular surgery or longstanding abnormal ventricular load:
- Previous VSD closure
- ToF repair (prolonged QRS duration is a risk marker)
- Pulmonary regurgitation and right ventricular enlargement
- Single ventricles
- Mustard or Senning repairs
- ccTGA.

Indications for ICD implantation in congenital heart disease are awaited.

General Considerations for the Treatment of Arrhythmias

- Obtain as much information on the patient as possible
- Assess the patient thoroughly for signs of heart failure and infection
- Obtain a 12-lead EKG and compare with previous EKGs (ACHD patients often have a broad QRS complex)
- Only transfer patients to a tertiary center once stable
- Seek expert advice early.

Syncope

Syncope is always a matter of concern in patients with congenital heart disease especially if they are cyanosed or have pulmonary hypertension.

Causes for syncope in ACHD

- Tachyarrhythmia
- Bradycardia from sinus node dysfunction, AV block
- Pulmonary embolism
- Severe pulmonary hypertension
- Severe obstructive lesion (valve stenosis, etc.)
- Aortic dissection, rupture
- Myocardial ischemia
- Hypotension (drug induced?)
- Vasovagal.

→ Any syncope in a patient with congenital heart disease should initiate thorough electrophysiological and hemodynamic assessment and ideally should involve an expert in the management of adults with congenital heart disease.

Heart Failure

In any patient with congenital heart disease presenting with heart failure, an acute underlying cause has to be excluded. The most common causes are:

- Arrhythmia
- Infection
- Ischemia

Adult patients with congenital heart disease often have very finely balanced hemodynamics with minimal cardiac reserve. Even minor changes in their condition can cause severe deterioration.

Lesions that present with left or systemic heart failure

- Left-sided valve disease (mitral and aortic valve)
- TGA after Mustard or Senning repair and ccTGA
- Systemic left ventricular dysfunction in older ToF patients.

Lesions that present with right or subpulmonary heart failure

- Fontan patients
- Pulmonary hypertension/Eisenmenger syndrome
- Right-sided valve disease (tricuspid and pulmonary valve)
- Mustard repair with obstruction of intra-atrial pathways
- Elderly patients with late repair or unrepaired ASD.

Table 15.1 Heart Failure Treatment—Considerations for ACHD Patients

	Pros	Cons
Loop diuretics	• Effective, improves symptoms	• Rapidly reduces preload • Caution in Fontan patients
Spironolactone	• Effective, improves symptoms	

ACE inhibitors	• Effective to reduce hypertension
	• Unknown long term benefits on heart function
		• Little evidence to improve heart function
		• Caution if
		  • Preload dependent
		  • Obstructive lesion present
		  • Renal dysfunction
		  • Pulmonary hypertension

Beta-blocker	• Anti-arrhythmic • Good for heart rate control	• Caution in bradycardia
Digoxin	• Rate control in atrial flutter	

Adapted from *Adult congenital heart disease: A practical guide.* Gatzoulis et al. (eds). 2005. BMJ Books, Blackwell Publishing Group (with permission).

Medical Treatment

Seek expert advice early.

- Find the cause
- Restore sinus rhythm as soon as possible in compromised patients
- Medical treatment will not affect anatomic lesions
- Treat with the standard therapies for heart failure, including diuretics, but be cautious with vasodilator therapy.

Glossary of Surgical Procedures

Arterial switch operation or Jatene procedure

This operation is for TGA patients. The surgeon performs a switch of the great arteries to bring the aorta in the former pulmonary artery position and the pulmonary artery in the former aortic position. The coronary arteries have to be transposed from the aortic root to the former pulmonary artery root (neo aorta). Ultimately, the left ventricle will perfuse the aorta and the right ventricle will perfuse the pulmonary artery.

Bentall operation

Replacement of the ascending aorta and aortic valve with a composite graft (conduit) and valve and re-implantation of the coronary arteries into the conduit.

Brock procedure

Palliative procedure for ToF patients. Closed resection of right ventricular musculature from the outflow tract using a biopsy-like instrument and dilatation (valvotomy) of the pulmonary valve.

Classic Blalock-Taussig (BT) shunt

Subclavian artery to ipsilateral pulmonary artery anastomosis (direct end-to-side junction).

Modified Blalock-Taussig (BT) shunt

Same shunt using a prosthetic graft.

Damus-Kaye-Stansel operation

This is surgery to connect the aorta and pulmonary artery in a side-to-side fashion to provide unrestricted blood flow from the systemic ventricle to the aorta. It is performed in patients with single ventricles and transposition of the great arteries and restrictive VSD leading to subaortic stenosis.

Fontan operation

Palliative operation for patients with 'single' ventricle physiology (p. 197). It involves diversion of the systemic venous return to the lung without interposition of a subpulmonary ventricle. It leads to volume unloading of the single ventricle and ideally to normalization of the arterial oxygen saturation.

Multiple variations of the procedure exist regarding the type of connection between the systemic veins and the pulmonary arteries:

- Classic Fontan: Connection between right atrium and pulmonary artery
- Extracardiac Fontan: Inferior vena cava connected to pulmonary artery via an extracardiac conduit combined with a Glenn shunt
- Bjoerk or RA-RV Fontan: Valved conduit between the right atrium and the right ventricle

Total cavopulmonary connection (TCPC): Inferior vena cava connected to pulmonary artery via an intra-atrial tunnel (also called lateral tunnel), combined with a Glenn shunt to the SVC.

Glenn shunt

Superior vena cava (SVC) to pulmonary artery anastomosis.

- Classical Glenn shunt: Anastomosis of the superior vena cava to the distal right pulmonary artery with ligation of the SVC below the anastomosis and division of the proximal right pulmonary artery from the pulmonary bifurcation
- Bidirectional Glenn shunt: Anastomosis of the superior vena cava to the undivided pulmonary artery.

Konno operation

This is a complex repair and reconstruction of the left ventricular outflow tract for patients with tunnel-like subvalvar left ventricular outflow tract obstruction. The operation involves enlargement of the outflow tract by inserting a patch in the interventricular septum and aortic valve replacement as well as enlargement of the aortic annulus and the ascending aorta.

Lecompte maneuver

Maneuver that brings the pulmonary artery in a position anterior to the ascending aorta (part of the arterial switch operation or Jatene procedure).

Mustard operation

Atrial switch operation for patients with TGA: redirection of the venous blood to the contralateral ventricle using pericardial or synthetic patches.

Norwood operation

Initial palliative procedure for the treatment of hypoplastic left heart syndrome with aortic atresia and hypoplasia of the ascending aorta. The operation involves the reconstruction of the neo-ascending aorta using the pulmonary valve and trunk and the creation of an aorto-pulmonary shunt (usually modified BT shunt).

Pott's anastomosis shunt

Descending aorta to left pulmonary artery anastomosis.

Rastelli operation

This is an operation for patients with TGA, VSD, and pulmonary stenosis. The VSD is closed in a way that the patch forms the left ventricular outflow tract to the aorta. The right ventricle is connected to the main pulmonary artery using a valved conduit.

Ross operation

This is aortic valve replacement by transplantation of the patient's pulmonary valve into aortic position (pulmonary autograft) and by replacing the pulmonary valve using a homograft valve. It has some major advantages:

- Potential of the neo-aortic valve (former pulmonary valve) to grow in children
- No need for anticoagulation.

Senning operation

Atrial switch operation for patients with TGA, redirection of the venous blood to the contralateral ventricle using the atrial wall and the septum.

Waterston shunt

Ascending aorta to right pulmonary artery anastomosis.

Chapter 16

Perioperative Care

207

Perioperative Issues

Each year, approximately 30 million individuals in the United States undergo noncardiac surgery. Approximately one-third have cardiac disease or major cardiac risk factors. Current estimated rates of serious perioperative cardiac morbidity vary from 1–10%. The incidence of perioperative myocardial infarction (MI) is increased 10- to 50-fold in patients who have risk factors or have had a previous coronary event.

The cardiovascular systems of patients who undergo general anesthesia and noncardiac surgical procedures are subject to multiple stresses and complications. A previously stable patient may decompensate postoperatively, leading to significant postoperative morbidity and mortality. The high number of cardiovascular complications reflects the nature of surgery: a stress test that cannot easily be stopped once the operation has started.

Pre-operative risk assessment is therefore an important element of informed consent and also influences the strategy for anesthesia and post-operative care. Collaboration between surgeons, anesthetists, and physicians, especially cardiologists, is essential to ensure optimal management.

Cardiac risk stratification allows clinicians to group patients into various risk categories; low-risk patients can be spared further testing, whereas intermediate- and high-risk patients should undergo preoperative investigations and treatment to reduce overall cardiac perioperative morbidity and mortality.

Preoperative Assessment

Medical opinion is sought on diagnosis, clinical status, and the appropriateness of the patient's current treatment. The medical opinion may conclude that further evaluation is required and/or recommend specific treatments, e.g. revascularization or pacing prior to surgery.

Guided by this medical opinion, the anesthetist can determine the patient's fitness for anesthesia and surgery and develop a strategy for anesthesia and post-operative care. This includes the extent of cardiovascular monitoring and the best location for post-operative care, e.g. intensive care or step-down unit. *Informed consent* will require consideration of the risks as well as the benefits of the procedure.

Predictors of Risk

The risk of perioperative cardiac complications relates to both the clinical status of the patient and the nature of the proposed surgery.

The following stratification of predictors is based on the American College of Cardiology/American Heart Association guidelines. Clearly, the highest risk occurs when a patient with a 'major' clinical risk factor(s) undergoes a 'major' risk surgical procedure.

Predictors Related to the Patient

Major

- Unstable coronary syndromes
- Acute or recent MI
- Unstable or severe angina (Canadian class III or IV p. 213)
- Decompensated heart failure
- Significant arrhythmias
- High grade atrioventricular block
- Symptomatic ventricular arrhythmias
- Supraventricular arrhythmias with uncontrolled ventricular rate
- Severe valvular disease.

Intermediate

- Mild angina (Canadian Class I or II p. 213)
- Previous MI (history, pathological Q waves)
- Compensated or prior heart failure
- Diabetes mellitus
- Renal insufficiency.

Minor

- Advanced age
- Abnormal EKG (left ventricular hypertrophy, LBBB, ST-T segment abnormalities)
- Rhythm other than sinus
- Low functional capacity (inability to climb one flight of stairs)
- History of stroke
- Uncontrolled systemic hypertension.

Special considerations

- Severe hypertension with target organ involvement, left ventricular hypertrophy, and strain
- Co-morbidity (not mentioned above)
- Obstructive airway disease
- Possible interactions between medication and anesthetic agents
- Most cardiovascular drugs can be safely administered throughout the perioperative period
- Angiotensin converting enzyme inhibitors and angiotensin receptor antagonists may have to be omitted on the morning of surgery to reduce the risk of intractable hypotension.

Predictors Related to Surgery

Major (reported cardiac risk >5%)

- Emergency major operation (particularly in the elderly)
- Aortic and other major vascular surgery
- Peripheral vascular surgery
- Anticipated prolonged procedures with large fluid shifts and/or blood loss.

Intermediate (reported cardiac risk generally <5%)

- Carotid endarterectomy
- Head and neck surgery
- Intraperitoneal and intrathoracic surgery
- Orthopedic surgery
- Prostate surgery.

Low risk

- Endoscopic procedures
- Superficial procedures
- Cataract surgery
- Breast surgery.

In addition, special consideration should be given to the following:

- Cardiovascular effect of aortic cross-clamping and de-clamping
- Gut handling leading to the release of inflammatory mediators
- Surgery likely to impair post-operative respiratory function.

Predictors Related to the Type of Anesthetic

There is a perception that in cardiac patients, spinal or epidural anesthesia is safer than general anesthesia. There is, however, no scientific evidence of reduced cardiac risk with these types of anesthesia. Where spinal or epidural anesthesia offers major advantages, monitoring needs to be extensive because of the possibility of rapid changes in vascular resistance due to autonomic blockade resulting in severe hypotension.

Local anesthesia and regional anesthesia (regional nerve blocks) are associated with a relatively low risk of post-operative cardiac events.

Determining Risk

Cardiac disease is not always clinically obvious, particularly where function is limited, e.g. by arthritis or peripheral vascular disease. Where potentially life-saving emergency surgery is required (e.g. ruptured aortic aneurysm, major trauma) it may be sufficient to identify risk and to anticipate and treat cardiac complications, with a view to further cardiac evaluation post-operatively.

In the non-emergency setting, patients with major clinical risk factors usually require further investigation and/or treatment. Broadly speaking, patients with no more than intermediate clinical risk factors, a functional capacity that would allow them to walk up a hill or play a round of golf, and who are undergoing surgery of intermediate risk or less can proceed with a low probability of cardiac events.

Where functional capacity is low and/or a major risk procedure is to be undertaken, it is reasonable to proceed to non-invasive functional investigation (e.g. exercise EKG, pharmacologic stress echo-cardiography, stress radio nuclide ventriculography, or stress perfusion scintigraphy). Low reserve increases substantially the risk of cardiac complications after major surgery and further evaluation (for example with a coronary angiography) may be indicated.

Need for Coronary Revascularization

Coronary artery bypass surgery or percutaneous coronary intervention may be necessary in selected patients to decrease the risk of cardiac complications from anesthesia and surgery. Current guidelines recommend that coronary revascularization, if indicated by conventional criteria (irrespective of planned non-cardiac surgery), should normally precede non-cardiac surgery. If coronary revascularization is not warranted for conventional clinical indications, revascularization should only be considered before high risk surgery (particularly major vascular surgery).

Perioperative Issues in Relation to Specific Conditions

Please read in conjunction with the patient-focussed approach (above).

Coronary Artery Disease

Coronary disease is the most frequent cause of cardiac complications from anesthesia and surgery. In susceptible individuals, coronary events may be precipitated by hemodynamic changes (tachycardia, hypotension, hypertension), perioperative hypoxemia (especially nocturnal hypoxemia after abdominal surgery), altered coagulation and post-operative anemia.

Angina
- Well-controlled angina increases the risk of anesthesia and surgery but this increase is generally acceptable

- Unstable angina is an absolute contraindication to elective surgery and must be investigated pre-operatively as morbidity and mortality are unacceptably high.

Prior myocardial infarction

- The time that has elapsed between MI and proposed elective surgery is important. An interval of 3–6 months is generally advocated. More recently a delay of only 6 weeks has been regarded as acceptable in uncomplicated MI with no ischemia on a stress test.
- Myocardial function is a major determinant of risk. Patients with low ejection fraction remain at high risk irrespective of the time that has elapsed since the acute infarction.

Prior CABG

Asymptomatic patients within 5 years of successful coronary revascularization are at low risk for perioperative cardiac events.

Prior PCI

Distant (>6 months) PCI should not adversely affect surgery. More recent PCI may be associated with risk for two principal reasons:

- In order to minimize the risk of stent thrombosis, patients usually receive aspirin and clopidogrel. The pronounced anti-platelet effect of these drugs poses a risk of hemorrhage and it is preferable to defer surgery until clopidogrel has been stopped for one week. When there is active bleeding or major emergency surgery is necessary, platelet transfusion may be given.
- Pro-thrombotic conditions associated with surgery can increase the risk of stent thrombosis. Therefore, where possible, it is generally preferred to defer surgery for 4 weeks after stent implantation. This should allow re-endothelialization of the stent without encroaching on the time window for re-stenosis. Consult with the interventional cardiologist prior to stopping clopidogrel when a drug-eluting stent was used.

Box 16.1 Prophylactic Perioperative Beta-blockade

Evidence of the efficacy of perioperative beta-blockade is mixed. In general, a patient should continue on beta-blockers for an established indication (for example, angina, hypertension, or an arrhythmia). There is some evidence that, particularly in patients undergoing high-risk vascular surgery, pre-treatment with beta blockers may reduce the risk of perioperative cardiac events. When possible, beta-blockers should be started days or weeks before elective surgery and the dose titrated to obtain a resting heart rate of approximately 60 beats per minute.

Table 16.1	Canadian Cardiovascular Society Classification of Angina
Class I	Symptom free for all normal activities. Angina with strenuous or prolonged effort.
Class II	Minor limitation. Symptoms with brisk effort on stairs, in the cold, or after meals.
Class III	Significant limitation of ordinary activity. Symptoms with one flight of stairs or walking on the flat at a normal pace.
Class IV	Any physical activity may provoke symptoms. Angina at rest.

Reprinted with permission from Goldman L, Hashimoto B, Cook EF, Loscalzo A: Comparative reproducibility and validity of systems for assessing cardiovascular functional class: Advantages of a new specific activity scale. *Circulation* 1981;64:1227–1234.

Arrhythmias

During anesthesia and surgery arrhythmias occur frequently and require treatment where there is evidence of hemodynamic compromise (including myocardial ischemia). See Chapter 8 (p. 75).

Arterial Hypertension

Hypertension confers a modest increase in the risk of cardiovascular complications of anesthesia and surgery irrespective of the admission blood pressure. A blood pressure greater than 180/110 requires treatment. However, the presence of target organ involvement is more important than the level of blood pressure.

Cardiac Failure

The patient's functional capacity is useful for predicting operative risk (see NYHA classification p. 67). The ability to climb one flight of stairs with some load (or equivalent) is considered adequate reserve for most surgeries. Heart failure management should be optimized before surgery.

Objective testing

- Echocardiography
- Radionuclide ventriculography (MUGA scan)
- Cardiac magnetic resonance.

Conduction Disorders

Pre-operative pacemaker insertion

The indications for pacemaker insertion are covered in Chapter 8, (p. 75). The current consensus is that in general, the indications for pre-operative pacemaker insertion, including temporary pacemaker insertion, are the same as those for the non-surgical setting. These include complete heart block, Mobitz type II block, and symptomatic bradycardia.

Valvular Heart Disease

Considerations the following in each case:

1. hemodynamic consequences
2. anticoagulation
3. risk of endocarditis
4. indirect considerations, e.g. arrhythmia, effects of LVH.

See also Chapter 9 on valve disease p. 109.

Hemodynamic

Severe aortic stenosis represents the most serious threat. This fixed obstruction to cardiac output permits very little adaptation when increased output is required. Peripheral vasodilatation, e.g. from regional anesthesia or hypotension from hemorrhage, cannot be matched by an adequate increase in cardiac output. The consequent fall in blood pressure can lead to coronary hypoperfusion, reduced myocardial function, and further hypotension. This is a potentially fatal downward spiral.

Even in **moderate aortic stenosis**, stiffness of the left ventricle reduces the tolerance of variability of filling conditions. In fluid overload, the left atrial pressure will increase sharply provoking pulmonary edema while low filling pressure (hypovolemia) or low diastolic filling time (high ventricular rates) will decrease cardiac output. Where symptoms or physical signs suggest aortic stenosis, a preoperative echocardiogram should be obtained.

Mitral stenosis. The onset of atrial fibrillation or loss of rate control will decrease diastolic filling and bring about a fall in cardiac output with a consequent increase in left atrial pressure. This can provoke an abrupt deterioration in functional class and may cause overt pulmonary edema.

Mitral and aortic regurgitation require careful fluid management and may benefit from afterload reduction, e.g. with nitrates and ACE inhibitors. In some cases it may be appropriate to alleviate valve lesions prior to surgery. Full discussion of valve interventions and their indications are given in Chapter 9 (p. 135 and 138). In considering intervention, the balance of risk must take into account the type of valve and the possibility of thromboembolic events or infective endocarditis related to future surgery.

Anticoagulation (p. 130)

- Mechanical prosthetic valves: Anticoagulation has to be discontinued before most surgeries. Warfarin is replaced by an intravenous infusion of heparin or low molecular weight heparin to facilitate pre- and post-operative anticoagulation. In emergencies, anticoagulation with warfarin can be transiently reversed by administration of fresh frozen plasma (FFP), which provides clotting factors

• Be very wary of giving vitamin K since this will prevent anticoagulation with warfarin for a prolonged period. With expert guidance, a small dose of vitamin K (e.g. 1 mg), can be administered.

Endocarditis Avoidance

Abnormal heart valves, prosthetic mechanical valves, or biological valves are at increased risk for infective endocarditis as organisms are introduced at the time of surgery.

A full discussion on the risks of bacteremia and on the nature and indications for prophylactic antibiotics is found in Chapter 9 (p. 116).

Keep vascular access to the minimum necessary. Take precautions to avoid infections at insertion. Observe the skin around lines for signs of infection and replace lines regularly. Seek to remove all vascular catheters as soon as they are no longer needed.

Pacemakers and Implantable Defibrillators

Establish the type of pacemaker or defibrillator, the indications for implantation and the functional settings from the patient's pacemaker identification card or from the center where it was implanted.

These devices are susceptible to electromagnetic interference (EMI). This can come from disparate sources but in the context of surgery, EMI from cautery equipment is the major concern. EMI may enter the device by direct electrical interference during cautery or exposure to an electromagnetic field (in which the device lead acts as an antenna). Bipolar leads, generally used in contemporary pacing systems, are much less sensitive to EMI than unipolar leads and therefore the likelihood of encountering perioperative EMI is exceedingly slim. EMI can result in:

• Inappropriate inhibition of paced output
• Asynchronous pacing
• Reprogramming (usually into a back-up mode)
• Defibrillators may interpret electrocautery as VF and deliver a shock.

Electrocautery is usually applied in unipolar configuration between the handheld instrument (cathode) and the anode attached to the patient's skin.

• Cautery should be avoided near the pacemaker/ICD generator
• Bipolar cautery should be used wherever possible.

Cardiac Surgery

The following is intended as a practical guide to situations commonly experienced after cardiac surgery.

Assessing the Hypotensive Patient Post Cardiac Surgery

Read the surgeon and anesthesiology notes. Was the operation straightforward? The surgeon will have noted any difficulties, e.g. where small caliber coronary arteries threaten graft patency, or problems with hemostasis. What was the pre-operative assessment of left ventricular function?

Note the blood pressure and pulse trends. Was there an abrupt change suggestive of an acute 'event' or has the change been gradual. Compare with pre-operative values. Determine peripheral perfusion. Is the patient cold and 'shut down' or peripherally vasodilated? What is the urine output?

Is the patient adequately filled? One size does not fit all in this respect. Patients with left ventricular hypertrophy but good LV systolic function (e.g. post aortic valve replacement) are likely to require higher filling pressures. In patients with significant tricuspid regurgitation (e.g. post mitral valve replacement), filling will be difficult to gauge from the venous pressure. Remember that early after surgery, you are likely to have the benefit of a CVP line (p. 31).

Does the EKG show evidence of myocardial ischemia? Has the rhythm changed? AF is common post-operatively (see opposite). New onset or fast AF may be sufficient to compromise blood pressure in susceptible patients.

Are the pericardial drains working? Has the rate of drainage changed (new bleeding, drain occlusion)? Hypotension with tachycardia, and elevated CVP may indicate pericardial tamponade. This can occur rapidly and may be caused by a relatively small volume of pericardial blood. Tamponade may reduce cardiac output due to its effects on filling. Post-operatively, this may be caused by localized effects on a single chamber. An urgent echocardiogram should be obtained. In extreme cases, sudden hemodynamic collapse necessitates emergency exploration and direct drainage with the chest reopened.

When hypotension persists despite correction of the reversible causes, further evaluation with echocardiography may be indicated. New wall motion abnormalities suggest perioperative infarction or 'stunning.' Consider support with inotropic drugs ± intra-aortic balloon pump. These measures are considered in greater detail in Chapter 4, (p. 21).

Atrial Fibrillation Post Cardiac Surgery

- AF occurs in approximately 25% of patients, and is more frequent in elderly patients and those with a prior history of AF
- If the patient is markedly compromised proceed to DC cardioversion (p. 256).
- Correct hypokalemia: keep K$^+$ at 4–5 mmol/L

- Most cases of post-operative AF are likely to return spontaneously to sinus rhythm, unless AF was present pre-operatively
- Control the rate with beta-blocker or digoxin
- Amiodarone IV (central line) may hasten reversion to sinus. In selected patients, continuation with oral therapy may be indicated
- Anticoagulation is needed if AF is persistent (begin with heparin and convert to warfarin)
- Outpatient review of continuing need for antiarrhythmic therapy and the need for cardioversion.

Atrioventricular Conduction Block Post Cardiac Surgery

- This is most likely after aortic valve surgery because of the valve's proximity to the AV node
- Pacing is necessary using epicardial pacing electrodes implanted during surgery, or a temporary transvenous system
- Permanent pacemaker implantation is often required. The need for a permanent pacemaker can be predicted by the following pre-operative features: AV block, LBBB, root abscess, calcified aortic annulus, aortic regurgitation, and prior MI.

Post-pericardiotomy Syndrome

This is an inflammatory (possibly autoimmune) pericarditis that occurs more than a week after cardiac surgery where the pericardium has been opened. The associated effusion may be serous or serosanguinous. It can be large and can lead to tamponade. It is often associated with fever, pericarditic pain, and malaise. The diagnosis is clinical. Echocardiography is helpful in determining the size, distribution, percutaneous accessibility, composition (e.g. fibrinous), and hemodynamic significance of the pericardial effusion. Treat with NSAIDs. The condition is usually self-limiting, but may recur.

Chapter 17

Cardiotoxic Drug Overdose

219

General Approach

Cardiovascular side-effects can occur with both cardiac and non-cardiac medication. In particular, side-effects secondary to recreational drug use are becoming more prevalent. Patient history may be unreliable and any witnesses should be sought.

General Management Principles

- Resuscitate the patient
- Consider the prevention of drug absorption:
- Activated charcoal (50 g orally) will absorb many drugs if given <1 hour after ingestion
- Gastric lavage can be considered if a substantial overdose has been ingested <1 hour previously. The evidence for benefit is weak and it is performed less commonly now
- Supportive care (e.g. airway maintenance, acid-base and electrolyte balance, treat seizures) is important
- Any unstable arrhythmias (VT, fast SVT >180/min) are better dealt with by cardioversion than drugs.

Further Help with Management

More detailed information and advice on patients is available at all times from members of the American Association of Poison Control Centers. Telephone advice is available at all times and is especially useful for complex cases or severe toxicity. The single telephone number 1-800-222-1222 directs the call automatically to the relevant local center.

Medical staff with specialist toxicology experience as well as physician-toxicologists are available for advice about seriously poisoned patients. The Poison Control Center can also advise about sources of supply for antidotes which are needed only occasionally and also about laboratory analytical services which may be helpful in the management of some patients.

Beta-blockers

There are large numbers of patients taking β-blocking agents and toxicity from accidental or deliberate overdose is therefore common. Over 15,000 cases are reported annually to poison control centers in the US, and the vast majority of these are accidental overdoses.

Mechanism of Toxicity

Beta-adrenoreceptor blocking agents act on cardiac (β_1) and non-cardiac (β_2) receptors. β_1-blockade causes bradycardia, hypotension, and decreased cardiac contractility. β_2-blockade results in broncho-constriction and hypoglycemia.

Toxic Dose

This is highly variable and depends on the clinical situation. Ingestion of two or three times the normal therapeutic dose may cause symptoms.

Presentation

Overdose with β-blocking drugs (e.g. propranolol, atenolol, labetolol, or sotalol) may cause rapid and severe toxicity with hypotension and cardiogenic shock. There is usually a sinus bradycardia, but sometimes the heart rate remains normal. Coma, convulsions, and cardiac arrest may occur. EKG changes include marked QRS prolongation and ST and T wave abnormalities. Sotalol can cause a prolonged QTc and VT, sometimes with torsades de pointes. Propranolol may cause bronchospasm in asthmatics and hypoglycemia in children.

Investigation

The diagnosis is clinical. Blood levels may be obtained, but will not be reported in time to aid diagnosis. Obtain an EKG and provide continuous cardiac monitoring. A bedside blood glucose level should be obtained, as well as baseline electrolytes and a complete blood count, since these are often required by the admitting teams.

221

Intervention

Monitor EKG, heart rate, and blood pressure, and give activated charcoal (1–2 mg/kg PO). Glucagon is the best treatment for severe cardiotoxicity or bronchospasm and seems to work by activating myocardial adenylcyclase in a way not blocked by ß-blockade. Glucagon 5–10 mg IV (50–150 µg/kg for child) usually produces a dramatic improvement in pulse and BP, with return of cardiac output and consciousness. Glucagon may cause sudden vomiting, which must be expected and the patient positioned appropriately. In severe poisoning, the benefits of glucagon may be transient and further doses or an infusion are needed (4 mg/h, reducing gradually). Some patients need a total of 50 mg of glucagon. Bradycardia and hypotension may respond to atropine (1–2 mg for adult; 0.02 mg/kg for child), but this is often ineffective. Bronchospasm may also be treated with β-agonists (e.g. albuterol). If glucagon is not available or is ineffective, use isoproterenol (5–10 µg/min) or dobutamine (2.5–10 µg/kg/min), increasing the dose as necessary depending upon the response. In cases of severe poisoning, discuss the case with the local poison control center. Cardiac pacing may be needed for bradycardia but is not always effective.

Differential Diagnosis

The following drugs also cause bradycardia and hypotension, and should be considered in the differential diagnosis:

- Calcium channel blockers
- Cyclic antidepressants
- Centrally-acting α-agonists
- Digitalis

Disposition and Documentation

Patients with bradycardia, hypotension, EKG changes, or altered mental status should be admitted to the ICU. Other patients should be observed for 6 hours, after which they may be discharged if they are ED patients and have remained asymptomatic. Document normal vital signs, a normal EKG, a normal blood glucose at the time of discharge, and the administration of charcoal. If the overdose is deliberate, a psychiatric consultation is required once the patient is medically cleared.

Calcium Channel Blockers

Calcium channel blockers are used in the treatment of a number of conditions such as angina, hypertension, and arrhythmias. The most common agents are diltiazem, nifedipine, and verapamil.

Mechanism of Toxicity

Blockade of the calcium channels found in both smooth muscle and myocardial cells leads to decreased smooth muscle tone and a lowered blood pressure, as well as a reduction in the heart rate. Calcium channel blockers have no effect on serum calcium levels.

Toxic Dose

Serious toxicity may occur even with ingestions slightly larger than the therapeutic dose.

Presentation

The presentation will depend on the amount ingested. The most common findings are dizziness, syncope, dyspnea, and confusion. Nausea and vomiting may also occur.

Investigation

Check the pulse (often slow and weak) and systolic blood pressure (usually <100 mmHg). Decreased perfusion will cause mental status changes and respiratory distress or pulmonary edema. Bradycardia

Table 17.1 Differentiating Calcium Channel Blocker Poisoning from Other Agents Causing Bradycardia and Hypotension	
Agent	Important Features in Overdose
Calcium channel blockers	Hyperglycemia is common Normal QRS width
Cholinergics (e.g. organophosphates)	Non-cardiac symptoms predominate: salivation, nausea, vomiting
β-blockers	Hypoglycemia common
Cyclic antidepressants	Wide QRS common

and AV block may lead to AV dissociation, with hypotension and cardiac arrest (especially in patients taking β-blockers). Obtain an EKG looking for AV block and ischemia. Metabolic acidosis, hyperkalemia, and hyperglycemia may occur, so obtain a complete blood count (looking for anemia) and electrolyte panel. Obtaining serum levels of calcium channel blockers has no role in therapy.

Intervention

- Give activated charcoal as soon as possible.
- Mild hypotension will usually respond to IV fluids.
- Give atropine (1–2 mg, child 0.02 mg/kg) for symptomatic bradycardia.
- For patients who remain with severe hypotension or bradycardia, give calcium chloride (e.g. 500 mg–1 g IV q10 minutes). This will reverse the prolonged intra-cardiac conduction. The dose may be repeated, and changed to a continuous infusion (e.g. 1 g/h) depending on the clinical response.
- Glucagon may help, as in β-blocker poisoning. Give 5–10 mg IV (50–150 μg/kg for child). However, if there is no response thus far, pacing may be needed.
- In patients refractory to all of the interventions above, inotropic support with dobutamine (2–20 mcg/kg/min), isoproterenol (2–10 mcg/min), or epinephrine (1–4 mcg/min of 1:10,000 solution) may be needed to maintain cardiac output.

Disposition and Documentation

Asymptomatic patients with a suspected overdose and those with mild symptoms of calcium channel blocker overdose should be observed for 6 hours or treated as above. If the symptoms improve, discharge (if in the ED) or psychiatric consultation (if indicated) is appropriate. All other patients should be admitted. Patients who have ingested a sustained-release preparation should be admitted to a monitored bed for continued observation.

Digoxin

Toxicity from the therapeutic use of digoxin, the most common cardiac glycoside, is relatively common, and an unintentional overdose is ten times more common than deliberate ingestion. Acute poisoning is rare, but may be fatal. Similar effects occur with digitoxin and very rarely with plants containing cardiac glycosides (such as foxglove and lily of the valley).

Mechanism of Toxicity

Cardiac glycosides inhibit the transport of sodium and potassium across the cell membrane. They also have a negative chronotropic action, from both vagal effects and a direct effect on the sinoatrial node.

Toxic Dose

Toxic effects may be noted with the ingestion of 1–3 mg of digoxin, but neonates and children are much less prone to the effects of overdose.

Presentation

The features will depend on whether the overdose was acute or chronic. Chronic accidental overdose is frequently seen in elderly patients. Patients present with a flu-like illness, nausea, vomiting, malaise, delirium, and xanthopsia (yellow flashes or discoloration of vision). Acute poisoning causes bradycardia with PR and QRS prolongation. There may be AV block, AV dissociation, and escape rhythms, sometimes with ventricular ectopics or ventricular tachycardia. Hyperkalemia occurs and in severe cases there is a metabolic acidosis due to hypotension and decreased tissue perfusion. The initial degree of hyperkalemia correlates with prognosis.

Investigation

Obtain a stat serum digitalis level, a stat potassium level and an EKG. The diagnosis is made by a history of ingestion and an elevated serum level of digoxin of greater than 2 ng/mL. Send a full electrolyte panel, since many patients on digoxin will also be on diuretic therapy, and a CBC. Check the serum magnesium and calcium levels since hypomagnesemia and hypercalcemia worsen the effects of digitalis toxicity. If a deliberate overdose is suspected, send a toxicology screen depending on your local protocol.

Intervention

The initial intervention is to provide supportive treatment, and monitor the EKG and vital signs. Then take the following steps:

- Give repeated doses of activated charcoal to reduce absorption and prevent the enterohepatic recycling of digoxin.
- Correct hyperkalemia above 5.5 mmol/L with sodium bicarbonate (1 meq/kg IV), glucose (e.g. one ampoule of D50) and insulin (0.1 unit/kg IV).
- Bradycardia and AV block are best treated with digoxin-specific antibodies. Resistant bradycardia should be treated with atropine (e.g. 1–2 mg IV). If atropine fails, cardiac pacing with a temporary pacer is needed but may be difficult since a high voltage is often needed for capture. VT may respond to lidocaine (1 mg/kg IV bolus followed by 1–4 mg/kg/min) or phenytoin (15 mg/kg IV at a rate less than 50 mg/min).
- Severe poisoning, evidenced by arrhythmias and hyperkalemia, is best treated with digoxin antibodies (Digibind®), which rapidly

correct the arrhythmias and hyperkalemia. The correct dose depends on an estimation of the size of the ingestion. Each vial of 40 mg will bind 0.5–0.6 mg of digoxin. If the actual size of the ingestion is known, use the following to determine the dose of digoxin-specific antibodies: Total number of vials = Amount of ingested digoxin (mg) × 2

• If the total amount ingested is not known, use the following table to guide initial therapy:

Acute Ingestion of Unknown Amount:	20 vials
Overdose from Chronic Therapy	6 vials

Disposition and Documentation

Digitalis has a half life of 30–50 hours and the peak effects may not occur for upto 12 hours post ingestion. Therefore, all patients with symptoms of digitalis overdose should be admitted for observation and therapy. Accidental overdose with normal serum digitalis levels may be discharged home after 8–10 hours of ED observation. Document your discussion with the PCP and the mechanism put in place to prevent a future accidental overdose.

Cyclic Antidepressants

Cyclic antidepressants were an important therapy for depression, but in recent years they have been largely (but not totally) replaced by the SSRI drugs. The number of overdose cases has declined as a result, and there are now fewer than one hundred deaths per annum from this class reported in the US. Amitriptyline is the most common drug in overdose.

Mechanism of Toxicity

TCA toxicity affects the central nervous and cardiovascular systems. Anticholinergic effects result in tachycardia and hypotension, as well as central effects such as somnolence, seizures or coma. Inhibition of the fast sodium channels results in myocardial depression and conduction disturbances.

Toxic Dose

This is variable, but is in the range of 20 mg/kg.

Presentation

Common features are tachycardia, dry skin, dry mouth, dilated pupils, urinary retention, ataxia, and drowsiness or coma. Unconscious patients often have a divergent squint, muscle tone and reflexes, myoclonus, and extensor plantar responses. The pupils are dilated and unreactive. In deep coma there may be muscle flaccidity with no detectable reflexes and respiratory depression requiring IPPV. Seizures occur in about 10% of unconscious patients and may precipitate cardiac arrest. Patients recovering from coma often suffer delirium and hallucinations and have jerky limb movements and severe dysarthria. Death may result from cardio-respiratory depression and acidosis.

Investigation

The earliest EKG finding is a sinus tachycardia. However, as the severity of poisoning increases the PR interval and QRS duration both increase. These changes help confirm the clinical diagnosis of cyclic poisoning in the unconscious patient. The P wave may be superimposed on the preceding T wave, giving the appearance of VT when the rhythm is actually sinus tachycardia with prolonged conduction. In very severe poisoning, ventricular arrhythmias and bradycardia may occur, especially in patients who are hypoxic. While a cyclic antidepressant level is obtainable, it does not necessarily correspond to the clinical severity of the ingestion, which should be based on clinical findings as EKG changes. However, a level greater than 1,000 ng/mL usually indicates a serious overdose.

Intervention

- Clear airway, intubate if necessary, maintain ventilation and give supportive treatment.
- Observe continuously, in view of the potential for rapid deterioration.
- Monitor EKG and check the SaO_2 especially in unconscious or postictal patients.
- Give activated charcoal by mouth or gastric tube if the airway is safe or can be protected. Further doses of charcoal may be required if a sustained release drug has been taken.
- Seizures should be treated in the usual way with lorazepam or diazepam IV.
- The mainstay of therapy is alkalinization and sodium therapy, which will reverse the cardiac effects and hypotension. Cardiac arrhythmias occur within a few hours of overdose and together with hypotension or QRS widening (greater than 100 milliseconds) are indications for sodium bicarbonate therapy. Give 2 meq/kg IV bolus of 8.4% sodium bicarbonate and repeat as needed. The usual initial adult dose is two 50 mL ampules, and children should get 1 mL/kg. The aim is to keep the serum pH between 7.45 and 7.55. Sinus tachycardia is common and does not itself require any intervention.
- Avoid all classes of antiarrhythmic drugs, since they will worsen the arrhythmia (due to sodium channel blockade) or hypotension.

- Correct hypotension by elevating the foot of the bed and giving IV fluids. Dopamine (2–10 μg/kg) is indicated for hypotension which remains unresponsive to usual therapies.
- Although once widely used, there is now no role for physostigmine, which may precipitate seizures and worsen arrhythmias and hypotension.

Disposition and Documentation

All patients requiring sodium bicarbonate should be rapidly admitted to the ICU. Patients with suspected cyclic overdose but without indications for sodium bicarbonate therapy should be treated with charcoal and observed on a monitor in the ED for 6 hours. If the patient remains asymptomatic after this period of time, she may be medically cleared and seen by a psychiatrist if indicated. Document the following:

- Normal vital signs.
- Normal EKG.
- Normal mental status.
- Negative toxicology screen for acetaminophen and salicylate overdose.

Follow-up plan after psychiatric consultation (if indicated).

Theophylline

Theophylline was once widely used to treat asthma, but is no longer used for this. As a result, many older patients, (but very few younger ones) with COPD or asthma are still treated with theophylline. Theophylline and aminophylline can cause fatal poisoning. Caffeine overdose presents in similar ways, but is less likely to cause seizures.

Mechanism of Toxicity

Theophylline releases catecholamines and stimulates β-receptors.

Toxic Dose

The therapeutic blood level is 15–20 mg/L. This level may be achieved with a single dose of 10 mg/kg. Ingestions of more than 50 mg/kg will result in serious toxicity. Toxicity may result from a single acute ingestion, or from chronic excessive doses are repeated. Symptoms of toxicity are usually noted at levels above 100 mg/L in acute overdose, but in acute-on-chronic overdose symptoms levels of only 20–30 mg/L may result in serious toxicity.

Presentation

The most common features are anxiety, tremor, nausea, vomiting, and tachycardia. There may be abdominal pain and hematemesis, increased muscle tone, hyperreflexia, and a headache or convulsions. Serious ingestion (resulting in levels above 100 mg/L) may present with seizures, ventricular arrhythmias, and hypotension. The seizures may become status epilepticus which is often very resistant to standard treatment. Many theophylline preparations are slow-release and may not produce serious toxicity for 12–24 hours after ingestion.

Investigation

Complex metabolic disturbances include a respiratory alkalosis followed by metabolic acidosis, hyperglycemia, and severe hypokalemia. In an acute overdose the hypokalemia is often profound, but this is rare in chronic ingestion. Obtain a serum theophylline level. Because of the use of slow-release preparations, the theophylline level should be repeated every four hours until a decline is noted. The diagnosis is made on the basis of an elevated serum theophylline level and the clinical findings described above.

Intervention

- Initiate supportive treatments: give oxygen and intravenous fluids, and take seizure precautions.
- Monitor heart rate and BP and obtain an EKG.
- Obtain venous access and measure a BMP, CBC, and plasma theophylline (which should be repeated after a few hours). Measure the potassium every 2–3 hours if the patient is symptomatic, since early correction of hypokalemia with IV potassium will help prevent dangerous arrhythmias. Remember that the hypokalemia represents a movement of extracellular potassium into the cells, and not a loss of potassium from the body. As theophylline levels drop, the potassium will shift back out, resulting in hyperkalemia. Treatment of hypokalemia must therefore be cautious and closely monitored.
- Perform gastric lavage if less than one hour has passed since ingestion. Give repeated activated charcoal, by NG tube if necessary.
- Intractable vomiting may respond to ondansetron (8 mg slowly IV in adult).
- Ongoing GI bleeding may require transfusion and ranitidine (but not cimetidine, which slows metabolism of theophylline).
- Tachycardia with an adequate cardiac output should not be treated. Non-selective ß-blockers (e.g. propranolol 1 mg IV up to a total of 10 mg) may help severe tachyarrhythmias and hypotension, but may cause bronchospasm in asthmatics.
- Control seizures with lorazepam or phenytoin. If the airway is at risk, rapid sequence intubation and IPPV should be initiated.

- Charcoal hemoperfusion or hemodialysis is reserved for those with signs of life-threatening toxicity, such as status epileptics, or arrhythmias. However, its use is controversial and best discussed together with your local Poison Control Center or toxicologist.

Disposition and Documentation

Patients with mild symptoms of overdose should be treated and observed in the ED for 6–8 hours. If their vital signs remain stable, and a repeat theophylline level shows a decline, discharge (or psychiatric consultation if indicated) is appropriate if there is a safe home environment. All other patients should be admitted.

Drugs Used in Cancer

A number of oncological therapeutic agents are known to be cardiotoxic. In the majority, these effects are cumulative, but a number of medications have acute cardiac side effects:

Interleukin-2

- Causes a capillary leak syndrome (hypotension, edema, effusions, arrhythmias)
- Stop infusion, administer steroids, antihistamines, and consider epinephrine.

5-Fluorouracil

- May cause myocardial ischemia and acute MI
- Stop 5-FU treatment and treat with conventional anti-anginal therapy.

Anthracyclines, e.g. doxorubicin, daunorubicin

- Chronic dose-related cardiomyopathy
- Arrhythmias.

Others

- Cisplatin   Acute myocardial ischemia
- Cyclophosphamide   Heart failure, hemorrhagic pericarditis
- Mitomycin C   Myocardial injury
- Vincristine   MI
- Vinblastine   MI
- Taxol   Bradycardia

Cocaine and Amphetamines

Cocaine and its derivative, 'crack,' are usually sniffed or smoked, but severe poisoning may occur in body packers or body stuffers. The cardiac features and management of amphetamine overdose are comparable to those of cocaine overdose (see above).

Mechanism of Toxicity

Cocaine is a local anesthetic and also causes central nervous system stimulation. It causes coronary artery vasoconstriction, which may result in angina or infarction.

Toxic Dose

Ingesting more than about one gram of cocaine is fatal. A line of snorted cocaine contains about 30 mg of cocaine. Individual tolerance is highly variable.

Presentation

Patients under the influence of cocaine present with varying degrees of euphoria, agitation, and tremulousness. There is often nausea or vomiting, and headache and hallucinations may occur. Seizures are common, and the patient may have been brought to the ED in a post-ictal state. Seek as much history as is possible from any friends or family, as well as the police or pre-hospital personnel.

Investigation

The pulse and blood pressure are usually very elevated. The pupils are dilated. Look for the signs of 'crack eye,' namely corneal abrasions and ulcerations from the heat and smoke of crack. There is often hyperpyrexia. Perform a careful physical exam looking for occult trauma (especially in patients in whom there is no history available), nasal septum perforation (following chronic snorting), and skin ulcers resulting from the injection of cocaine. Once the patient is cooperative, obtain an EKG looking for ischemia or tachyarrhythmias. In cases of suspected co-ingestion send a toxicology screen. Send serum electrolytes looking for evidence of renal failure, and a creatinine kinase to exclude rhabdomyolysis. In cases of suspected head injury obtain a CT scan, since following the patient's mental status is not reliable. If body packing is suspected obtain a plain abdominal X-ray.

Intervention

The first priority in patients who are agitated is to ensure your own safety and that of the other staff and patients in the ED. Call security and apply your restraints policy in all cases where there is a concern the patient's behavior is putting him or others in danger.

- Maintain a clear airway and adequate ventilation.
- Give activated charcoal if cocaine has been ingested within the last hour.
- To control seizures and agitation give lorazepam (2 mg IV) or diazepam (5 mg IV) repeated as needed. Do not be surprised that large amounts are often needed.

- If hypertension is severe, give nitroglycerin (e.g. 5 mcg/min IV and increase as needed). Another alternative is a calcium channel blocker (e.g. diltiazem 20 mg IV over 2 minutes).
- Avoid ß-blockers; they will allow unopposed stimulation of cardiac α-receptors, resulting in worsening hypertension or ischemia.
- Treat chest pain which appears to be of cardiac origin as you would any patient with ischemic symptoms (see p. 42). Patients are at greatest risk of myocardial ischemia in the first hour following cocaine ingestion, when cocaine blood levels are at their highest. Start with oxygen, sublingual NTG, aspirin, and morphine. If this fails to help, apply NTG to the chest wall or start an intravenous infusion. Benzodiazepines are also helpful in treating ischemic type pain (see above). If the EKG suggests an acute MI, treat as appropriate for that condition (see p. 49).
- Phentolamine is an α-blocking agent that reverses cocaine-induced coronary artery vasoconstriction. It is rarely used, because the measures above are usually sufficient. However, in ischemia non-responsive to the usual measures, consider giving phentolamine (start with 2 mg IV and repeat every 5 minutes as needed).
- Hyperpyrexia requires cooling and sedation with benzodiazepines.
- Smoking cocaine may result in pharyngeal burns, due to the hot gases and anesthetic action of cocaine. Intubation may be needed to protect the airway from worsening edema.

Body Packers and Body Stuffers

Body packers swallow condoms filled with cocaine in order to smuggle it across a border. Once at their destination, they take laxatives to collect the condoms. Body stuffers are those dealers who are forced to swallow packages of cocaine, usually when they are about to be apprehended by police. Both are at very high risk of toxicity should the packages or condoms erode. Minimally symptomatic patients should be treated with charcoal followed by whole bowel irrigation. Obtain a plain abdominal X-ray to look for the packages and estimate their number. All patients should be admitted to the hospital until all the packages have safely passed. Clinical symptoms of toxicity which cannot be easily controlled should prompt a rapid surgical consultation to remove the packages in the operating room.

Disposition and Documentation

Patients with cocaine intoxication usually respond rapidly to ED interventions. Mild symptoms of intoxication should be treated and observed in the ED for 6 hours. If the mental status returns to baseline and there is no evidence of end organ damage, the patient should be discharged. Document a repeat EKG at the end of the ED stay which shows no ischemia, a normal BUN and creatinine, a normal creatinine kinase, and a normal urinalysis. Give the patient referral options for local drug-rehabilitation facilities. Patients with evidence of renal damage, ongoing ischemia, rhabdomyolysis, or hyperthermia should be admitted to the hospital.

Ecstasy

'Ecstasy' (3,4-methylenedioxymetamphetamine, MDMA) is an amphetamine derivative which is used as an illegal stimulant drug. It is taken orally as tablets or capsules, or occasionally in powder form. Other amphetamines (such as MDA and MDEA) have similar effects. These drugs are often diluted and contaminated with other toxic compounds.

Mechanism of Toxicity

MDMA causes the release of both catecholamines and serotonin within 30 minutes of ingestion. Its effects last between 2 and 6 hours.

Toxic Dose

The toxic dose is highly variable, depending on the formulation of the drug. Symptoms are generally seen with the ingestion of 1–2 mg/kg, and hyperthermia is noted with the ingestion of more than about 5 mg/kg.

Presentation

Patients typically present with paranoia and impaired reasoning. They are agitated and may complain of a headache, muscle pains, nausea, and vomiting. They are often diaphoretic, with dilated pupils and nystagmus. The vital signs will show a tachycardia, and the body temperature is often elevated. There is usually an initial hypertension followed later by hypotension. In severe cases, there may be heat stroke with hyperthermia, muscle rigidity, seizures, coma, rhabdomyolysis, cardiac arrhythmias, and eventual renal failure.

Investigation

The diagnosis is made on the history of ingestion and the clinical findings. A standard urine toxicology screen will detect other co-ingestants as well as amphetamines, but levels are not helpful for clinical management. The urine should also be tested for blood and myoglobin, since rhabdomyolysis is often seen. A serum toxicology screen should also be sent if co-ingestants are suspected. Obtain a bedside blood glucose to check for hypoglycemia. Send a serum metabolic panel to look for hyponatremia. Although it is unusual, massive ingestion may cause DIC and hepatitis, so it is a reasonable to send LFTs and a PT/INR. An EKG should be obtained (to exclude cyclic antidepressant co-ingestion which widens the QRS complex), and patients should be monitored because of the risk of cardiac arrhythmias.

Intervention

- Maintain a clear airway and adequate ventilation.
- Maintain aspiration precautions.
- Give oxygen by nasal cannula or face mask.
- Correct hyperthermia with fans, cool water mist, ice packs, or a cooling blanket. If these measures fail, give dantrolene (1 mg/kg IV, repeated if necessary up to 10 mg/kg in 24 hours).
- Give oral activated charcoal, by NGT if necessary.
- Treat agitation or seizures with lorazepam (e.g. 2 mg IV repeated as needed) and add phenytoin (15 mg/kg IV) if the seizures continue.
- Provide reassurance to the patient and if possible, place the patient in a quieter part of the ED.
- Correct hypotension, dehydration, and rhabdomyolysis with IV fluids.
- For severe hypertension, give esmolol (500 µg/kg IV bolus over one minute, followed by 50 µg/kg/min IV, titrated as needed) or phentolamine (2–5mg IV).

Disposition and Documentation

Patients with mild symptoms of overdose should be treated and observed in the ED for 6 hours. If their mental status improves, discharge (or psychiatric consultation if indicated) may be appropriate if there is a safe home environment. Patients with seizures, rhabdomyolysis, or continued mental status changes should be admitted.

Drug-induced QT Prolongation

Many factors influence acquired QT prolongation, including genetic susceptibility (separate from congenital long-QT syndromes), metabolic state (including hypokalemia and hypomagnesemia), other concomitant drugs, and heart rate. Thus the emergence of QT prolongation relies not just on the drug ingested, but on a combination of this and many predisposing factors. The occurrence with any particular drug is therefore unpredictable, but several drugs have been shown to be associated:

The main risk is of polymorphic VT (Torsade de Pointes) (see p. 102).

Table 17.2 Some Causative Drugs	
Class 1a antiarrhythmics:	Quinidine, procainamide, disopyramide
Class 1c antiarrhythmics:	Flecainide
Class III antiarrhythmics:	Sotalol, amiodarone, dofetilide
Tricyclic antidepressants:	Amitryptiline, imipramine, clomipramine
Psychotropic agents:	Lithium, chlorpromazine, haloperidol
Antihistamines:	Terfenadine, loratidine
Antimicrobials:	Erythromycin, clarithromycin, quinine, chloroquine, ketoconazole
Immunosuppressants:	Tacrolimus
Recreational drugs:	Cocaine

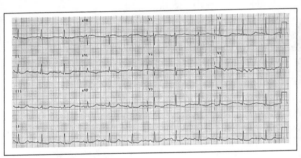

Figure 17.1 Drug-induced long QT.

Presentation

Common presentation of a prolonged QT are recurrent dizziness or syncope and palpitations. Patients may also present with polymorphic ventricular tachycardia (Torsade de Pointes). This is a rare form of polymorphic VT, associated with hypomagnesemia, hypokalemia, and a long QT interval. This long interval may be congenital or drug related (e.g. sotalol, antipsychotics, antihistamines, antidepressants). A constantly changing electrical axis results in QRS complexes of undulating amplitude.

Investigations

The diagnosis is made on EKG, which will show a prolonged QT interval. Other EKG presentations are VT and Torsade de Pointes. Check the serum electrolytes (especially K^+, Mg^{2+}, Ca^{2+}).

Intervention

For patients in Torsades, treat with IV magnesium sulfate (5 mL of 50% over 30 minutes). Refractory cases may require overdrive pacing.

The first intervention in a stable patient is to identify and withdrawing the offending drug. Avoid empirical antiarrhythmic therapy, and the concurrent use of agents that prolong QT interval and/or inhibit hepatic cytochrome P450 isoenzyme (e.g. fluoxetine) should be avoided.

Chapter 18

Miscellaneous Conditions

Hypertensive Emergencies

A *hypertensive crisis* (previously called malignant hypertension) occurs in <1% of patients with hypertension. Severe prolonged elevation of blood pressure (diastolic >130 mmHg) can result in end-organ damage, mostly affecting the central nervous system, kidneys, and cardiovascular system. Prognosis depends on the degree of end-organ damage, rather than the level of the blood pressure. Survival rate has improved considerably and >90% of patients are alive at 1 year.

Presentation

- Angina, left ventricular failure
- Headache, visual disturbance, irritability, altered consciousness, seizures. (When this occurs it is referred to as hypertensive encephalopathy.)
- Nausea and vomiting
- In the setting of aortic dissection
- Hematuria or acute renal failure
- In association with catecholamine excess (pheochromocytoma, recreational drug overdose)
- During pregnancy with eclampsia/pre-eclampsia.

Clinical Signs

- Check blood pressure in both arms (consider aortic dissection) and in the legs (consider coarctation)
- Fundoscopy (retinal hemorrhages, exudates, or papilledema)
- Full neurological examination (focal abnormalities)
- Examine for renal bruits (consider renal artery stenosis).

Investigations

- 12 lead ECG
- Chest X-ray
- CBC (microangiopathic haemolytic anemia), electrolytes
- Urinalysis
- Further laboratory investigations (according to working diagnosis) include cardiac troponin, thyroid hormones, urine collections for catecholamines.

Management

ED patients with hypertensive emergencies should be admitted to hospital for bed rest and monitoring. The aim of blood pressure management is to lower systolic pressure by 10% in the first hour and then by a further 15% in the next few hours. Treatment can begin with a beta-blocker (e.g. atenolol) or long acting calcium antagonist (e.g. amlodipine). IV antihypertensive therapy may be required if oral therapy is not effective. Commonly used agents are nitrates, nitro-prusside, and labetalol (see p. 148).

Hypertensive Emergencies in Specific Conditions

- *Aortic dissection* (see p. 144). A more rapid reduction in blood pressure is required with a target systolic pressure of <120 mmHg. Start with esmolol 1 mg/kg IV bolus over 30 seconds followed by 50–150 mcg/kg/min IV infusion.
- Patients with *subarachnoid hemorrhage* should be treated with IV sodium nitroprusside (0.2–0.5 mcg/kg/h and titrate as need). To control vasospasm give nimodipine 60 mg po (or via NGT in unconscious patients)
- Patients with *pheochromocytoma* should be treated with the alpha-blocker phentolamine (2–5 mg intravenously), followed by beta-blockade if necessary. The risk of beta-blockade is of unopposed alpha-adrenoreceptor stimulation
- In *pregnancy* some anti-hypertensive drugs are contraindicated. See p. 180 for specific advice
- *Cocaine* abuse may precipitate a hypertensive emergency (p. 229). Intravenous benzodiazepines and vasodilator therapy are recommended
- Hypertension caused by *monoamine oxidase inhibitors* should be managed with benzodiazepines and with a short-acting antihypertensive such as sodium nitroprusside.

Further Management

A combination of beta-blockers, calcium channel blockers, ACE-inhibitors, and other antihypertensives are often necessary to normalize blood pressure.

Traumatic Heart Disease

Blunt Cardiac Trauma

- Usually occurs as a result of motor vehicle accidents, crush injuries, falls, prolonged cardiopulmonary resuscitation
- Injuries range from myocardial bruising to fatal cardiac rupture
- Non-fatal injury usually results in sub-epicardial or myocardial bruising
- Investigations for blunt cardiac trauma are:
  - EKG-T wave changes (non-specific) or conduction abnormalities (bundle branch block)
  - Cardiac enzymes can be elevated (though not believed to be prognostically important)
  - Echocardiography may show regional wall motion abnormalities or a pericardial effusion

• Management is bed rest, monitoring, and analgesia. Complete recovery is the rule.

Commotio cordis
A cause of sudden cardiac death, particularly in young men with no underlying cardiac disease. Impact to the precordium (usually from a baseball or other hard object) over the center of the left ventricle just before the onset of the T wave is believed to cause VF and sudden death.

Penetrating Cardiac Trauma
Obtain an emergent cardiothoracic consultation in all cases of penetrating cardiac trauma.

• Stab and gunshot wounds are the most common causes and usually affect the right and left ventricles (anterior structures)
• A large proportion of stab wounds to the heart present with pericardial tamponade, whereas gun shot victims usually present with shock due to hemorrhage
• Immediate ultrasonography is indicated and if a pericardial effusion is visible in an unstable patient, urgent cardiothoracic intervention is required
• Pericardiocentesis is discouraged in acute trauma. The blood clots quickly and may be difficult to remove
• Do not remove a knife or other penetrating instrument unless instructed to do so by a cardiothoracic surgeon.

Cardiac Tumors

Primary cardiac tumors are rare. Secondary malignant deposits in the heart are more common. Three-quarters of primary cardiac tumors are benign and the majority of these are myxomas. Diagnosis is by echocardiography, MRI, and CT imaging.

Clinical Features
• Cardiac symptoms and signs related to obstruction (dyspnea from pulmonary venous congestion and pulmonary edema, syncope)
• Signs of systemic embolization (stroke, peripheral emboli p. 172)
• Systemic or constitutional symptoms (fever, weight loss, fatigue)
• Arrhythmias (due to direct infiltration of the conduction tissue or myocardial irritation).
→ Cardiac tumors are the great mimickers.

Benign Tumors
Cardiac myxomas
Represent 50% of cardiac tumors. Rare forms are multiple (LAMB and NAME syndromes) and inherited (autosomal dominant). Usually

present around age 50. Most commonly arise in the atria from the fossa ovalis. Left atrium > right atrium. Symptoms and signs (clubbing, rash, 'tumor plop'—similar to 3rd heart sound) similar to endocarditis, malignancy and collagen vascular disease. Blood test may reveal anemia, a raised CRP, and a low ESR. Echocardiography is normally diagnostic. Myxomas generally have a broad base but some are pedicled. Management is urgent surgical excision. Follow-up echocardiography is required as inadequate excision can lead to recurrence.

Papillary fibroelastomas

Often detected as small incidental lesions on the aortic and mitral valve. Fragments may embolize leading to coronary or cerebral obstruction. Surgery is generally indicated to improve prognosis but small right-sided lesions may be monitored.

Others

- Rhabdomyoma (most common primary cardiac neoplasm in children)
- Fibroma (most commonly resected childhood tumor)
- Hemangiomas
- Cardiac lipomas
- AV nodal tumors (small cystic mass—a cause of sudden cardiac death).

Malignant Tumors

Sarcomas

Extremely rare. May occur in any part of the heart but most commonly involve the right atrium. Includes angiosarcoma, osteosarcoma, leiomyosarcoma, rhabdomyosarcoma. Management is with a combination of surgery, chemotherapy, and radiotherapy. Outcome is generally poor with median survival less than 1 year.

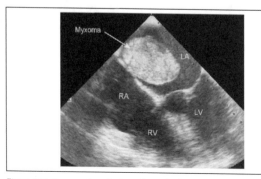

Figure 18.1 Transesophageal echocardiography demonstrating a large myxoma attached to the septum between the right atrium (RA) and left atrium (LA).

Cardiac lymphoma
Radiological staging is required to distinguish between primary cardiac lymphoma and generalized lymphoma. Management is usually with chemotherapy.

Metastatic cardiac tumor
Tachycardia, arrhythmias, heart failure in a patient with carcinoma should raise the suspicion. May present with pericardial effusion and/or tamponade. Associated malignancies include malignant melanoma, leukemia, lymphoma, and carcinoma of the stomach, liver, colon, rectum, and ovary.

Chapter 19

Procedures

General Considerations

There is Always Time to Think

There are very few emergencies that require an *immediate* response. A focused period of reflection and planning, supported when required by the opinion and contribution of others, is an essential prelude to the successful performance of a practical procedure—especially in the demanding setting of an acute clinical problem.

Is the Proposed Procedure Indicated?

This may seem an odd first question but it is the correct starting point. Many a practical procedure is abandoned after prolonged or multiple fruitless (and often painful) attempts with an observation to the patient that 'We can do without it.' Consider the indications for the proposed procedure and any special factors that may affect the likelihood of success or the objective risk. Review all alternative approaches to the problem. Commit to a procedure only if the intervention is considered essential or has much to offer, at a risk judged acceptable to you *and* your patient. A process of informed consent is ideal but may not be possible or appropriate in certain clinical settings.

Do You Have the Skills to Perform the Procedure?

It is your professional duty to act within the bounds of your established competence. Never hesitate to ask for help or guidance or to initiate a referral to an appropriate consultant. This text aspires to serve as a practical *aide-memoire* and is not a substitute for formal training and practical experience. Even if experienced and confident in a procedure, never underestimate the role and importance of assistants or other professionals (e.g. radiographers in temporary pacing).

Do You Have the Setting and Equipment for the Procedure?

If you are still in residency, inform your more senior resident of your intention and schedule

- Secure time, free of likely interruption
  - Are there any competing urgent clinical concerns?
- Rearrange the room and furniture to secure optimum access
  - Adjust patient position, bed height, and remove obstructions
- Ensure adequate lighting
- Prepare and check all items of equipment that will be required
- For complex or unfamiliar procedures, perform a mental rehearsal to establish the sequence of your planned action and as a checklist for the equipment requirements

244

- Ensure compatibility of interdependent items. Will the pacing wire fit through the venous access line? Will the pacing wire fit to the pacing box?
- Prepare in advance items that do not demand sterile handling, e.g.
  - Infusions for central venous lines
  - Transducers and monitors for pressure lines.

Central Venous Lines

Choice of Approach
The three main approaches to central venous cannulation are:
1. internal jugular vein
2. subclavian vein
3. femoral vein

You should aim to become familiar with at least two of these routes.

General Points—Applicable to All Approaches

- Pay attention to sterility to minimize infection risk. Prepare the skin and drape with sterile dressings. Wear sterile gloves and a gown.
- The patient should be positioned with head-down tilt. This fills the central veins, increasing their available size for cannulation and minimizes the risk of air embolization during the procedure.
- Whenever possible use the Seldinger (guidewire through needle) technique. Catheters over needle devices (similar to peripheral IV cannulae) are more difficult to place.
- Mount the needle on a syringe containing a few mL of 0.9% saline.
- Position the guidewire on the sterile field but within easy reach.
- Advance the needle, maintaining negative pressure by aspiration.
- If the vein is not entered, withdraw the needle slowly, maintaining syringe aspiration. Sometimes the needle transfixes the vein and cannulation is only evident on slow withdrawal.
- After an unsuccessful pass:
  - Flush the needle to remove debris that may clog its lumen.
  - Reassess the anatomical landmarks and identify a modified line for the next attempt. Explore the region systematically.
- When the needle enters the vein and blood is aspirated, be prepared to make minor adjustments (advance or retract) to ensure free flow of blood.
- Fix the needle with one hand and carefully remove the syringe.

- Pass the flexible end of the guidewire down the needle. The wire should pass with minimal resistance. Passage can sometimes be facilitated with minor rotation of the wire or needle (to change the angle of the bevel).
- If resistance persists remove the wire and check the needle position by aspiration with a syringe. When half of the wire is in the vein, remove the needle and place the cannula and its dilator over the wire. Do not advance the sheath into the body until a short length of wire is visible protruding from the distal end of the dilator and is secured with a firm grasp.
- If there is resistance to insertion of the cannula, consider enlarging the skin nick. If there is resistance in the deeper layers (e.g. clavipectoral fascia for subclavian lines) it may be necessary to first advance a dilator of smaller caliber (without its sheath) to open the track.
- Once the line is in place, remove the dilator and secure the cannula with suture and a transparent occlusive dressing.
- Radiographic examination (penetrated films) can be used to check the line position but this investigation should not preclude emergency use of a line following uncomplicated insertion.

The Internal Jugular (IJ) Approach

This has emerged as the most common route for central venous access. When compared to subclavian access, the IJ approach has a reduced risk of pneumothorax and allows compression hemostasis if bleeding occurs. The line, once placed, may be more uncomfortable for patients and there may be an increased tendency for displacement of temporary pacing wires introduced via this access. The right IJ is preferred to the left as it avoids the thoracic duct.

- Prepare and drape the skin
- Identify the apex of the triangle between the clavicular and manubrial heads of sternomastoid (see Figure 19.1)
- Infiltrate the skin and subcutaneous tissue with lidocaine 1–2%
- Nick the skin with a small (e.g. Number 11) scalpel blade
- Palpate the line of the carotid artery and insert the needle lateral to this line at an angle of 45° to the skin, aiming for the right nipple area (or anterior superior iliac spine)
- The vein is superficial and cannulation should be achieved at a depth of a few centimeters. Do not advance beyond this as the apex of the lung could be injured.

The Subclavian Approach

The subclavian approach allows access to the patient if the area around the patient's head is unavailable (for example during a cardiac arrest). A line inserted by this route lies on the anterior chest, is

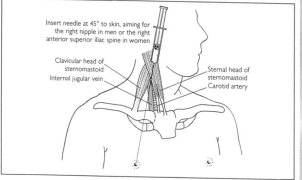

Insert needle at 45° to skin, aiming for the right nipple in men or the right anterior superior iliac spine in women

Clavicular head of sternomastoid

Internal jugular vein

Sternal head of sternomastoid

Carotid artery

Figure 19.1 Internal jugular central line insertion.

comfortable for the patient, and easy to manage. The main limitations of the approach are a risk of pneumothorax and an inability to apply pressure to the target vessels in the event of multiple venous or inadvertent arterial puncture.

- Prepare and drape the skin
- Identify the junction between the medial third and lateral two-thirds of the clavicle. This is usually at the apex of a convex angulation as the clavicle sweeps laterally and cranially
- The skin incision point is 2 cm inferior and lateral to this point
- Infiltrate the skin and subcutaneous tissue at this point and up to the edge of the clavicle at the first landmark
- Move the needle tip stepwise down the clavicle, infiltrating local anesthetic. Keep the needle horizontal until it moves below the clavicle
- Prepare the cannulation needle and follow the same initial track as the anesthetic needle
- When the needle lies just below the clavicle swing the needle round to aim at the nadir of the suprasternal notch
- Keeping the needle horizontal and parallel to the bed (avoiding lifting the hands off the body and angling the needle tip down) minimizes the risk of pneumothorax.

Femoral Vein Approach

The femoral approach allows easy cannulation of a large vein and is valuable in an emergency setting. The area can be compressed in the event of bleeding and temporary pacing can be achieved by this route. The main limitations relate to subsequent patient immobility and a probable increased risk of line infection.

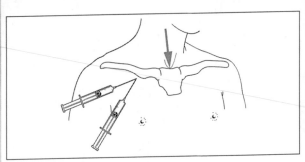

Figure 19.2 Right subclavian vein central line insertion.

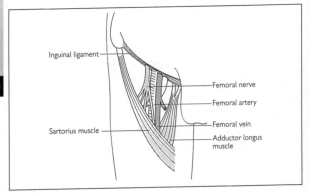

Inguinal ligament

Femoral nerve

Femoral artery

Femoral vein

Sartorius muscle

Adductor longus muscle

Figure 19.3 Right femoral vein anatomy.

- The patient should be lying flat with the leg slightly adducted and externally rotated
- Shave the groin, prepare the skin, and drape
- Palpate the femoral artery below the inguinal ligament, over or slightly above the natural skin crease at the top of the leg
- The femoral vein lies medial to the femoral artery
- Infiltrate local anesthetic at the skin surface and deeper layers
- Advance the cannulation needle at 30–45° to the skin surface
- The vein usually lies ~2–4 cm from the skin surface.

Pulmonary Artery (PA) Catheters

The main purpose of PA (e.g. Swan-Ganz) catheters is to monitor intracardiac pressures. Other, more specialized, catheters allow the calculation of indices of cardiac function and vascular resistance. Ensure that the correct equipment is available and prepared including the pressure transducers and monitors.

- Connect the patient to EKG monitoring and insert a peripheral IV cannula.
- Secure central venous access using a sheath designed to allow the introduction of PA catheters.
- Prepare the PA catheter by flushing the lumens—usually labeled distal, mid, and proximal, describing the exit lumen in the catheter. Most PA catheters include a soft balloon, inflated with air and designed to encourage floatation of the catheter tip (with blood flow), through the right heart and into the pulmonary vasculature. Test this balloon with an inflation/deflation cycle.
- Attach real time pressure monitoring to the distal channel of the PA catheter and insert the catheter to a depth of 8–10 cm.
- Inflate the balloon to encourage flow through the right heart. Deep inspiration can encourage passage across the tricuspid valve.
- Progress of the catheter can be assessed with X-ray screening but the more usual method is to observe the characteristic waveforms (see figure opposite) recorded in the right atrium, ventricle and in the pulmonary artery. The right ventricle is usually gained at a catheter length of 25–35 cm and the PA at 40–50 cm.
- Ventricular ectopics and non-sustained VT may occur during passage (usually indicating that the catheter is in the right ventricle) but do not demand treatment in the absence of circulatory collapse.
- Do not continue to advance the catheter if there is no progress. This risks knot formation with catheter coiling in a chamber. Deflate the balloon, withdraw to the right atrium, and attempt another passage. In patients with low cardiac output or established right heart pathology it may be necessary to pass the catheter under fluoroscopy.
- When in the pulmonary circulation, advance the catheter tip to a position where the wedge pressure can be measured when the balloon is inflated. Deflation of the balloon between readings minimizes the risk of trauma or rupture of a pulmonary vessel.
- A good wedge tracing exhibits a classic left atrial pattern with 'a' and 'v' wave morphology (see figure opposite). It is lower or equal to the PA diastolic pressure and has no dicrotic notch (seen in most PA tracings). The wedge pressure usually fluctuates with respiration. If the pressure tracing is damped and tends to increase in a ramp fashion this implies 'overwedging' and partial balloon deflation or catheter withdrawal may be required.

Right heart pressure tracings

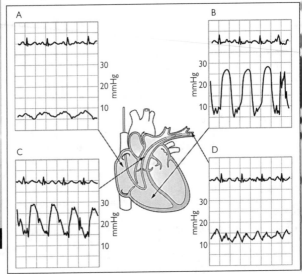

Figure 19.4 Right heart catheterization.
In each panel, the EKG is shown at the top with the corresponding pressure trace from the distal port of a PA catheter at the bottom. The characteristic pressure traces indicate the position of the catheter as it traverses the right heart. Record the pressures obtained from each location and the systemic arterial blood pressure.
A: Right atrial pressure trace in sinus rhythm. Atrial pressure is clearly lower than that of RV or PA. The 'a' wave coincides with atrial contraction while the 'v' wave reflects atrial filling against the tricuspid valve (closed during RV systole). The 'a' wave will be absent in atrial fibrillation. Large 'v' waves are indicative of tricuspid incompetence.
B: The right ventricular pressure trace is characterized by large swings in pressure that correspond to RV contraction and relaxation.
C: In the PA, the systolic should be equal to RV systolic (in the absence of right ventricular outflow tract obstruction or pulmonary stenosis). Note the dicrotic notch corresponding to closure of the pulmonary valve.
D: Pulmonary capillary wedge pressure. With the PA catheter balloon inflated, the distal port is insulated from the right heart and it is effectively exposed to left atrial pressure. In the absence of pulmonary embolism or pre-capillary pulmonary hypertension, PA diastolic pressure should approximate closely to PCWP.

Table 19.1 **Normal Ranges**		
RA	0–8 mmHg	
RV	systolic 20–25 mmHg	diastolic 6–12 mmHg
PA	systolic 20–25 mmHg	diastolic 4–8 mmHg
PCWP	6–12 mmHg	

Temporary Pacing

Consider drugs or external pacing as a means of immediate support if required.

Transvenous Temporary Pacemaker Insertion

- Insert a peripheral IV cannula and connect an EKG monitor (avoid external wires that will be visible when screening with X-rays)
- Using full sterile precautions, secure central venous access with a sheath of larger diameter than the temporary wire to be used. If subsequent permanent pacing is a possibility, try to leave at least one subclavian venous access untouched
- Under X-ray screening, advance the wire into the right atrium. The wire has a J-shaped distal contour which allows the tip to be directed by rotation of the proximal end of the wire
- Direct the wire towards the apex of the right ventricle (this lies just medial to the apex of the cardiac silhouette on AP screening)
- If the wire does not move directly over the tricuspid valve it may be necessary to form a loop of wire in the atrium, usually achieved with the tip on the right lateral atrial border. Rotation and advancement of the wire may then result in prolapse through the tricuspid valve
- As the wire enters the ventricle, some ectopic activity is usual and helps confirm a ventricular position
- The wire can inadvertently enter the coronary sinus. Its orifice lies above the tricuspid valve. A wire in the coronary sinus appears more cranial on AP screening and on a lateral view moves posterior (rather than the desired anterior direction of a right ventricular lead)
- Manipulate the wire so that the tip curves downwards to the apex of the ventricle. In its final position the line of the wire should resemble the heel of a sock in the right atrium (see Figure 19.6), with the toe in the apex of the right ventricle
- Connect the lead to the pacing box and test the threshold for capture. Pace at a rate above the intrinsic cardiac rate while slowly turning down the box output (start at 3 V). The EKG monitor is observed to identify the output at which capture is lost. Increase again slowly to recapture. This is the pacing threshold. A threshold of ≤1 V is desirable. Output is set to at least 3× the pacing threshold

251

- Test the stability of the lead position by observing lead motion and the ability to pace the heart during deep inspiration and coughing
- Suture the lead and sheath to the skin and apply transparent occlusive dressings
- Secure the external portion of the lead with tape or other fixatives. Fixing a loop on the skin should mean that inadvertent tugs on the wire will tighten the loop rather than pulling out the wire.

External (transcutaneous) Temporary Pacing

With gel pads at the apex and right parasternal position, set the rate to 70/min in demand mode. Turn up the output until electrical capture and confirm output with pulse. Note that uncomfortable skeletal muscle contraction will occur and may result in EKG artifact. Sedation is usually required.

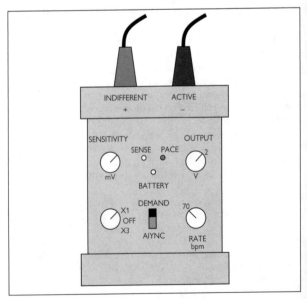

Figure 19.5 Standard controls for an external pacemaker.

Box 19.1 Configuring the Pacemaker Settings

Set to DEMAND at a RATE of, e.g. 70 beats per minute. The pacemaker will, on a beat to beat basis, PACE when it does not detect ventricular activity above that rate. The red PACE light will illuminate on each occasion. When the spontaneous ventricular rate is above the pacemaker rate, the box will inhibit and the red SENSE light will illuminate. An OUTPUT set to at least 3× pacemaker threshold will ensure that each impulse 'captures' the ventricle. The SENSITIVITY should be adjusted to ensure that each intrinsic beat is detected but that skeletal muscle interference does not lead to pacemaker inhibition (the lower the setting, the more sensitive the pacemaker).

- Note that instigating pacing may lead to pacemaker dependence.
- Ensure that the pacemaker is set to DEMAND. Asynchronous pacing risks inducing ventricular arrhythmias.

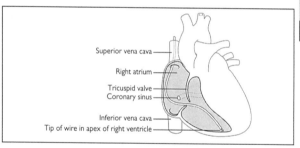

Figure 19.6 Temporary pacing wire position.

Inserting an Arterial Line

Although the femoral and brachial arteries can be used, the best approach is via the radial artery. This is a superficial vessel, easily palpated at the wrist, medial to the radial styloid. In the vast majority of people, a dual blood supply to the hand (via the ulnar artery and palmar arch) ensures adequate distal limb perfusion even if the radial artery is occupied by a catheter or closes by subsequent thrombosis.

- Revise the general considerations for venous line insertion (p. 244)
- Position the patient's hand with the palm upwards. Place a support (bandage roll or 500 mL fluid bag) to support the lower forearm and allow the wrist to rest in passive extension
- Prepare and drape the wrist
- Infiltrate local anesthetic at the skin surface and subcutaneous layer

- Use a special radial artery catheter pack with small caliber needle, guide wire, and cannula
- Palpate the radial pulse
- Aim to cannulate proximal to the flexor skin creases to avoid the tough flexor retinaculum
- Advance the needle at 45° to the skin. As the artery is entered, blood flow is observed from the needle hub
- Other aspects of the cannulation follow the pattern of central venous line insertion
- Secure the cannula and attach a pressure monitoring line, transducer, and flush facility.

Pericardiocentesis

Emergency drainage of the pericardial space is usually performed for the management of cardiac tamponade. When known or suspected tamponade has created a cardiac arrest situation, the procedure can and should be performed as an immediate and potentially life-saving measure. In other, less critical cases, echocardiography should be performed first. This investigation allows confirmation of the diagnosis and provides important information about the wisdom of and approach to pericardial aspiration.

Aspiration should only be attempted if there is a substantial fluid collection (>2 cm separation) between the pericardial layers at the access point of intended drainage. Following cardiac surgery or with certain chronic and infective etiologies, there can be localized tamponade of a cardiac chamber, not amenable to percutaneous drainage. In these cases consult with cardiothoracic surgery.

Imaging during the procedure is recommended. A cardiac catheterization laboratory is the ideal environment with radiographic screening and pressure monitoring, though echocardiographic imaging is increasingly used. These options may be not be available to critically ill ED patients who require emergent pericardiocentesis. Conscious sedation may be used if time and the patient's condition allow.

Procedure
- Position the patient at 45° to encourage pooling of the effusion at the inferior surface of the heart
- Prepare the skin and drape the patient in a sterile fashion
- Infiltrate local anesthetic along the drainage track (passing just under the costal margin, following a line towards the tip of the left scapula)
- The skin incision point lies just below the xiphisternum. Use a scalpel blade to make a small incision to reduce skin friction for the passage of the drainage catheter
- Advance the needle, with syringe attached, maintaining negative pressure, and observe for the aspiration of fluid

- If echocardiography is used, agitated saline may be used to confirm the presence of the needle in the pericardial space
- Remove the syringe when fluid is obtained and advance the guidewire through the needle so that it loops in the cardiac shadow on X-ray screening or is visible in the pericardial space with echocardiography
- Remove the needle, leaving the guidewire in place
- Advance a dilator over the wire. Several passes may be required
- Advance the catheter over the wire and into the pericardial space
- Fluid can now be aspirated with a syringe
- Symptoms and hemodynamic compromise in tamponade will improve with removal of modest volumes of fluid (e.g. 20–50 cc)
- Samples are sent for biochemical, immunological, and microbiological analysis
- The drainage bag can then be connected, secured with sutures at the skin entry point, and dressed with transparent occlusive dressings
- The catheter is usually left in situ for several hours to gauge the rate of drainage or re-accumulation (judged by echocardiography).

Box 19.2 Key Items of Equipment

A number of manufacturers now supply pericardial drainage packs.

- Long needle (15 cm) of at least 18 G calibre. A short bevel is an advantage to avoid potential cardiac laceration
- 'J' tip guidewire (0.035" diameter)
- Dilator (5–7 French)
- Pigtail or other drainage catheter with multiple distal side-holes
- Large caliber syringe for aspiration
- Drainage bag and connecting tubing

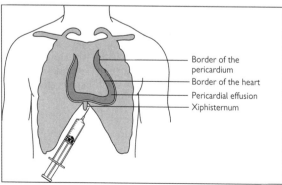

Border of the pericardium
Border of the heart
Pericardial effusion
Xiphisternum

Figure 19.7 Pericardiocentesis.

Cardioversion/Defibrillation

The quickest and most effective method of restoring sinus rhythm.

- Cardioversion is traditionally performed under sedation with intravenous benzodiazepines or under general anesthesia (typically with propofol) according to your local hospital protocol
- Full resuscitation, airway management, external pacing facilities, and trained personnel should be immediately available
- Ensure that the patient is well oxygenated, has not eaten for at least 4 hours (unless an emergency) and for elective procedures, patients should have signed a consent form
- As a minimum, monitoring should include indirect arterial oxygen saturation, blood pressure, and EKG monitoring
- Ensure the defibrillator electrodes are connected firmly to the machine, connect the EKG leads of the defibrillator to the patient and select a lead with the tallest QRS complex.

Ventricular Arrhythmias

- Place gel electrode contact pads over the sternum and at the apex of the heart
- Defibrillation for VF should be performed as quickly as possible using unsynchronized high initial energies (200–360 J monophasic, 150–200 J biphasic)
- If defibrillation is repeatedly unsuccessful then check the device settings and consider a different defibrillator
- Cardioversion of hemodynamically stable VT is usually performed under sedation with intravenous benzodiazepines
- If the patient is hemodynamically deteriorating do not delay in order to wait for an anesthesiologist. If there is time use sedation (e.g. midazolam 2–10 mg IV), ensuring close airway and respiratory monitoring
- Ensure the defibrillator is set to 'synch' so that the defibrillation shock is timed to coincide with the R wave. A dot should appear on the R wave of the EKG (and not the T wave). Use different leads if the synchronization is not optimal. Typical starting energies for the cardioversion of VT are 200 J monophasic and 150 J biphasic.

Atrial Arrhythmias (AF and Atrial Flutter)

External direct current (DC) cardioversion for AF has a success rate of 70–90% for restoring sinus rhythm. Since as little as 5% of the energy delivered externally actually reaches the heart, high external energies have to be used. Monophasic defibrillators deliver energy in one direction, whereas modern biphasic devices deliver the energy wavefront across the heart in two directions. The success rate for cardioversion using a biphasic defibrillator is higher than for mono-phasic devices.

- For elective cardioversion, it is vital to know the patient's anticoagulation status before cardioversion. If the international normalized ratio (INR) has been greater than 2.0 for at least 4 weeks, the risk of thromboembolism for elective cardioversion of AF is less than 1%
- It is also useful to know the serum K^+ before defibrillation, as hypokalemia may precipitate early reinitiation of AF
- Place gel electrode contact pads over the sternum and at the apex of the heart
- Ensure the defibrillator is set to 'synch' so that the defibrillation shock is timed to coincide with the R wave. A dot should appear on the R wave of the EKG (and not the T wave). Use different leads if the synchronization is not optimal
- Higher initial energies are more likely to restore sinus rhythm for AF (360 J monophasic, 200 J biphasic). Lower energies (200 J monophasic, 150 J biphasic) are suitable for atrial flutter
- Firm pressure on the defibrillator electrodes (8–12 kg) significantly improves the cardioversion success rate by reducing thoracic impedance
- If sinus rhythm has not been restored after two shocks at maximum output consider changing the electrode position to anteroposterior by either rolling the patient onto their right side or by positioning an electrode plate behind the patient
- If sinus rhythm is still not restored after an anteroposterior shock then the patient should be recovered in the left lateral position and an alternative strategy considered (such as internal cardioversion or drug facilitation), usually at a later date.

Chapter 20

EKG Library

The following collection of EKGs is presented to act as a reminder of the 12-lead EKG patterns of common (and a few uncommon) cardiac conditions.

Right Bundle Branch Block

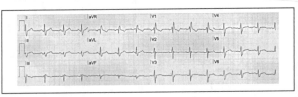

Figure 20.1 RBBB.
Broad QRS complex with an RSR pattern in V1 ('M' shape) and an S wave in V6 ('W' shape). There is also 1° AV block.

Trifascicular Block

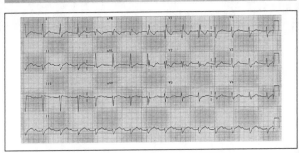

Figure 20.2 There is right bundle branch block, 1° AV block and left anterior hemiblock (left axis deviation).

Junctional Rhythm

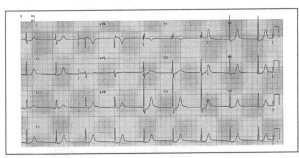

Figure 20.3 P waves are seen before the first complex but then are buried within the QRS complex. p. 78.

Second Degree Heart Block (Mobitz I)

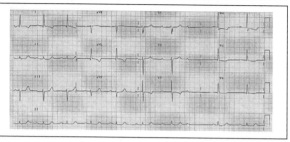

Figure 20.4 There is progressive lengthening of the PR interval until a P wave is non-conducted and a QRS is dropped (Wenckebach). The PR interval after the dropped beat is the shortest. p. 81.

Complete Heart Block

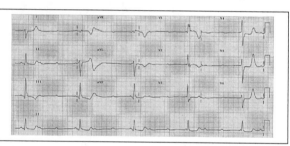

Figure 20.5 There are regular non-conducted P waves with a broad complex QRS escape rhythm. There is no association between the atrial and the ventricular rates. Management p. 81.

Atrial Fibrillation

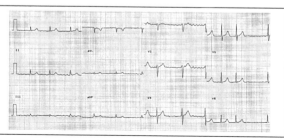

Figure 20.6 Irregularly irregular ventricular rhythm with no discernible P waves. Management pp. 87–89.

Pre-excited Atrial Fibrillation

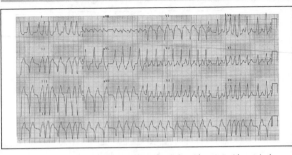

Figure 20.7 An irregular broad complex tachycardia with very rapid ventricular activation and conduction. Management p. 90.

Atrial Flutter

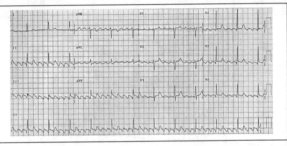

Figure 20.8 The baseline is irregular with a 'saw-tooth' pattern. The flutter waves are conducted with a 4:1 pattern to the ventricle. Management p. 90.

Atrial Tachycardia

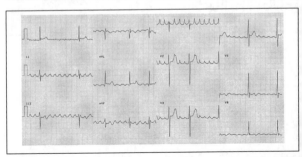

Figure 20.9 The baseline is irregular with very rapid atrial activation (300 bpm) and a positive P wave in V1 suggesting a focal atrial tachycardia. The baseline returns to normal between each atrial beat. Management p. 94.

Supraventricular Tachycardia (AVNRT)

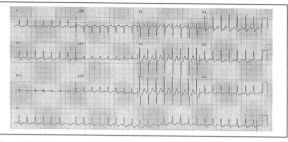

Figure 20.10 A narrow complex tachycardia.
The terminal deflection upon the R wave of the complexes of V1 is likely to represent the R-prime (R') sign. R' suggests a terminal portion of P wave is inscribed there. With a ventricular-to-atrial conduction time so short, AVNRT is the most likely diagnosis. Management p. 95.

Supraventricular Tachycardia (AVRT)

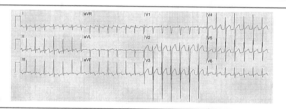

Figure 20.11 A narrow complex tachycardia.
There is retrograde P wave activation (clearly seen in V1 before the QRS complex). Management p. 95.

Pre-excitation

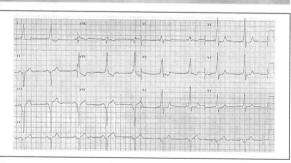

Figure 20.12 Short PR interval due to the presence of a delta wave. There is a RBBB-type pattern present, suggesting the accessory pathway is left sided. The negative delta waves inferiorly suggest that the accessory pathway is posteroseptal. Management pp. 83–84.

Ventricular Tachycardia

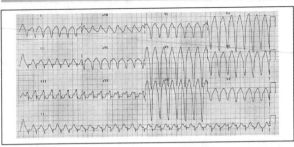

Figure 20.13 A broad complex tachycardia with a ventricular rate of 180 bpm. AV dissociation is seen with buried P waves in V6. There is concordance across the chest leads. Management p. 271.

Accelerated Idioventricular Rhythm

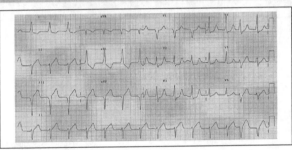

Figure 20.14 An automatic ventricular rhythm with a rate <100 bpm. Usually seen in the context of myocardial ischemia or infarction.

Long QT

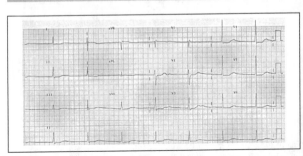

Figure 20.15 The QT interval (start of the Q wave to the end of the T wave) is prolonged (>600 ms). p. 102.

Brugada Syndrome

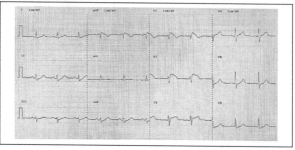

Figure 20.16 Right precordial ST elevation with T wave inversion in V1–V3. Association with sudden cardiac death. p. 20.

Arrhythmogenic Right Ventricular Cardiomyopathy

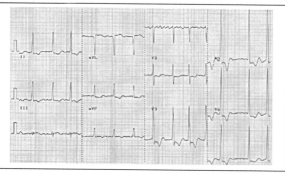

Figure 20.17 T wave inversion is seen in the right precordial leads (V1–V3). There is an epsilon wave (a small spike representing a late right ventricular potential) seen in V1 and V2 in the upstroke of the ST segment. Associated with VT. p. 100.

Pacemaker Lead Failure

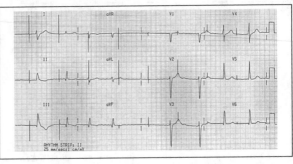

Figure 20.18 Pacemaker spikes can be seen with no ventricular capture. The ventricular lead had displaced.

Cardiopulmonary Resuscitation

Advanced Cardiac Life Support (ACLS) Protocols

The protocols below are the most recent recommendations of the American Heart Association.

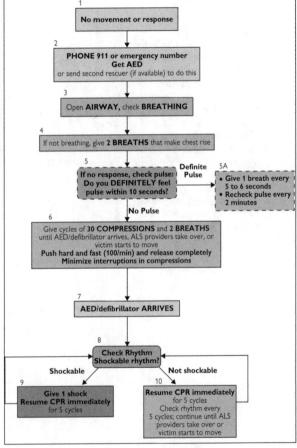

Figure 21.1 Adult BLS Healthcare Provider Algorithm.
Reprinted with permission 2005 AHA Guidelines for Cardiopulmonary Resuscitation and Emergency Cardiovascular Care, Part 4: Adult Basic Life Support. *Circulation.*2005;112: IV-19-IV-34. © 2005, American Heart Association, Inc.

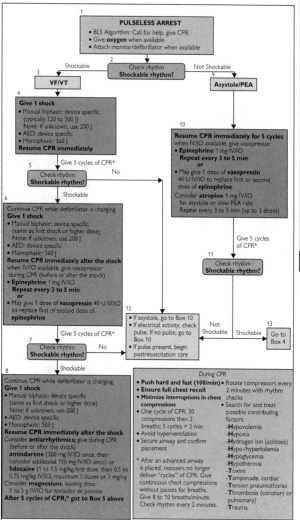

Figure 21.2 ACLS Pulseless Arrest Algorithm.
Reprinted with permission 2005 AHA Guidelines for Cardiopulmonary
Resuscitation and Emergency Cardiovascular Care, Part 7.2: Management of Cardiac
Arrest. *Circulation.*2005;112: IV-58-IV-66. © 2005, American Heart Association, Inc.

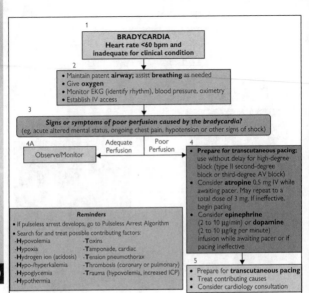

Figure 21.3 ACLS Bradycardia Algorithm.
Reprinted with permission 2005 AHA Guidelines for Cardiopulmonary
Resuscitation and Emergency Cardiovascular Care, Part 7.3: Management of
Symptomatic Bradycardia and Tachycardia. *Circulation*.2005;112: IV-67-IV-77.
© 2005, American Heart Association, Inc.

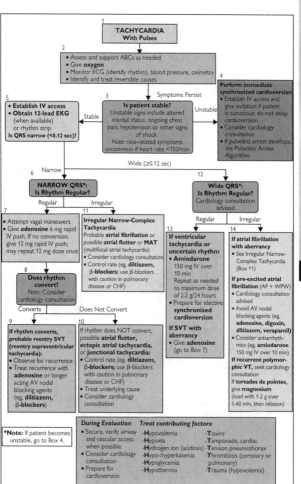

Figure 21.4 ACLS Tachycardia Algorithm.
Reprinted with permission 2005 AHA Guidelines for Cardiopulmonary
Resuscitation and Emergency Cardiovascular Care, Part 7.3: Management of
Symptomatic Bradycardia and Tachycardia. *Circulation*.2005;112: IV-67-IV-77.
© 2005, American Heart Association, Inc.

Pediatric Advanced Cardiac Life Support (PALS) Protocols

The protocols below are the most recent recommendations of the American Heart Association.

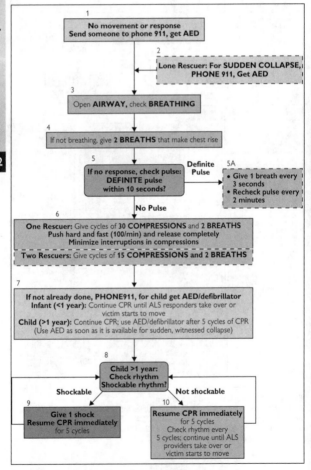

Figure 21.5 Pediatric Healthcare Provider BLS Algorithm.
Reprinted with permission 2005 AHA Guidelines for Cardiopulmonary Resuscitation and Emergency Cardiovascular Care, Part 11: Pediatric Basic Life Support. *Circulation*.2005;112: IV-156-IV-166. © 2005, American Heart Association, Inc.

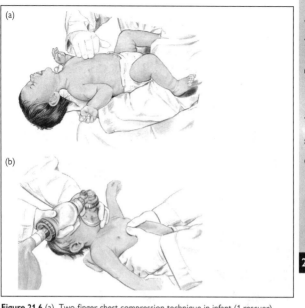

Figure 21.6 (a) Two-finger chest compression technique in infant (1 rescuer).
(b) Two thumb–encircling hands chest compression in infant (2 rescuers).

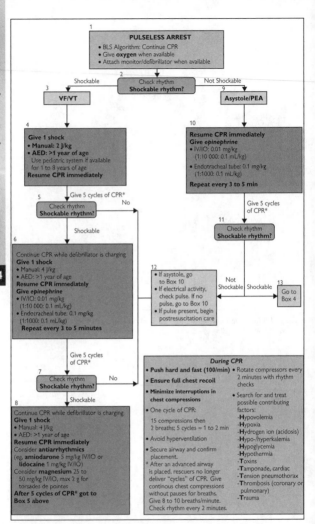

Figure 21.7 PALS Pulseless Arrest Algorithm.
Reprinted with permission 2005 AHA Guidelines for Cardiopulmonary
Resuscitation and Emergency Care, Part 12: Pediatric Advanced Life Support.
*Circulation.*2005;112: IV-167-IV-187. © 2005, American Heart Association, Inc.

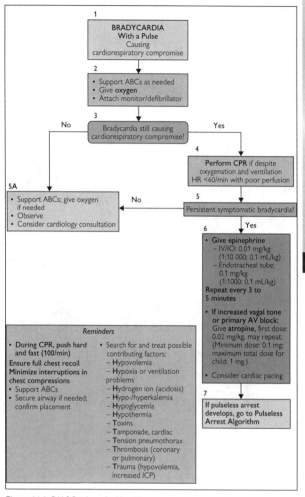

Figure 21.8 PALS Bradycardia Algorithm.
Reprinted with permission 2005 AHA Guidelines for Cardiopulmonary
Resuscitation and Emergency Care, Part 12: Pediatric Advanced Life Support.
*Circulation.*2005;112: IV-167-IV-187. © 2005, American Heart Association, Inc.

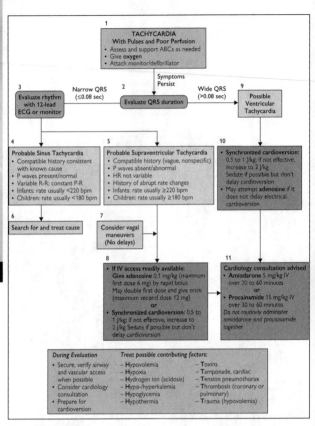

Figure 21.9 PALS Tachycardia Algorithm.
Reprinted with permission 2005 AHA Guidelines for Cardiopulmonary
Resuscitation and Emergency Care, Part 12: Pediatric Advanced Life Support.
*Circulation.*2005;112: IV-167-IV-187. © 2005, American Heart Association, Inc.

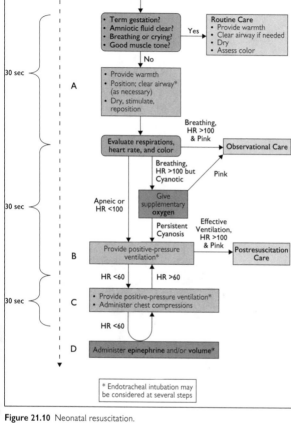

Figure 21.10 Neonatal resuscitation.
Used with permission of the American Academy of Pediatrics, 2005 AHA
Guidelines for Cardiopulmonary Resuscitation and Emergency Cardiovascular
Care. *Circulation* 2005;112: IV-188-IV-195.

Index

Page numbers with "*f*" and "*t*" denote figures and tables, respectively.